DRUG MISUSE AND COMMUNITY PHARMACY

DRUG MISUSE AND COMMUNITY PHARMACY

Edited by

Janie Sheridan

School of Pharmacy, The University of Auckland, New Zealand

and

John Strang

National Addiction Centre, Institute of Pyschiatry at the Maudsley Hospital, London

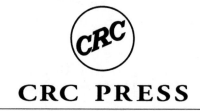

CRC PROTECT
CRC PRESS

Boca Raton   London   New York   Washington, D.C.

Library of Congress Cataloging-in-Publication Data

Catalog record is available from the Library of Congress

Visit the CRC Press Web site at www.crcpress.com

© 2003 by CRC Press LLC

No claim to original U.S. Government works
International Standard Book Number 0-415-28290-X PB
0-415-28289-6 HB
Printed in the United States of America   2 3 4 5 6 7 8 9 0
Printed on acid-free paper

Contents

Contributors

Dr Stuart Anderson
Senior Lecturer
Department of Public Health and Policy
London School of Hygiene and Tropical Medicine
London UK

Constantine Berbatis
Lecturer
School of Pharmacy
Curtin University of Technology
Perth
Australia

Professor Virginia Berridge
Professor of History
Department of Public Health and Policy
London School fo Hygience and Tropical
  Medicine
London UK

Professor Christine M Bond
Professor of Primary Care
Department of General Practice and
  Primary Care
University of Aberden
Aberdeen
UK

Max Bulsara
Biostatistician
Department of Public Health
University of Western Australia
Australia

Gihan Butterworth
Formerly of Addiction Services
Maudsley Hospital
London
UK

Dr Emily Finch
Consultant Psychiatrist and Honorary Senior
  Lecturer
National Addiction Centre
Institute of Psychiatry/Maudsley Hospital
London

Dr Glenda F Fleming
Laision Development Manager (Pharmacy)
Research and Development of Office for the
  Health and Personal Social Services in
  Northern Ireland
Belfast
UK

Dr Chris Ford
General Practitioner
Lonsdale Medical Centre
London
UK

Christine Glover
Member of Council
Royal Pharmaceutical Society of
  Great Britain
London
UK

Dr Laurence Gruer
Consultant in Public Health Medicine
Public Health Institute of Scotland
Glasgow
UK

Dr Robert Hill
Clinical Psychologist
Addictions Services
The Bethlem Royal Hospital
Beckenham
Kent
UK

Dr Carmel M Hughes
Senior Lecturer in Primary Care Pharmacy and
    National Primary Care Scientist
School of Pharmacy
The Queen's University of Belfast
Belfast
UK

Dr Francis Keaney
Clinical Research Worker and Honorary Specialist
    Registrar
National Addiction Centre
Institute of Psychiatry/Maudsley Hospital
London
UK

Dr Catriona Matheson
Senior Research Fellow
Department of General Practice and
    Primary Care
University of Aberdeen
Aberdeen
UK

Professor James C McElnay
Professor of Pharmacy Practice and
    Head of School of Pharmacy
School of Pharmacy
The Queen's University of Belfast
Belfast
UK

Dr Sile O'Connor
Addiction Pharmacist
Formerly of School of Pharmacy and Addiction
    Research Centre
Trinity College
Dublin
Ireland

Dr Tara Rado
Clinical Psychologist
Addictions Services
The Bethlem Royal Hospital
Beckenham
Kent
UK

Kay Roberts
Area Pharmacy Specialist – Drug Misuse
Greater Glasgow Primary Care NHS Trust
Glasgow
UK

Associate Professor Janie Sheridan
Associate Professor of Pharmacy Practice
The University of Auckland
Formerly of National Addiction Centre
Institute of Psychiatry/Maudsley Hospital
London
UK

Dr Trish Shorrock
Senior Pharmacist
Leicester Community Drug Team
Leicester
UK

Professor John Strang
Professor of the Addictions
National Addiction Centre
Institute of Psychiatry/Maudsley Hospital
London
UK

Professor V Bruce Sunderland
Professor and Head of School
School of Pharmacy
Curtin University of Technology
Perth
Australia

Dr David J Temple
Director of Pharmacy Continuing Education
The Welsh School of Pharmacy
Cardiff University
Cardiff
UK

John Witton
Health Services Research Co-ordinator
National Addiction Centre
Institute of Psychiatry/Maudsley Hospital
London
UK

An introduction to the book: context, aims and definitions

Janie Sheridan and John Strang

Two decades ago there probably would have been no need for a book which described the role and involvement of community pharmacy in services for drug misusers. Some community pharmacists would have been in contact with drug misusers through the dispensing of a small number of methadone prescriptions, or through furtive requests for injecting equipment, but there was no defined role for working with drug misusers. However, with the increasing numbers of individuals injecting drugs and the advent of HIV, community pharmacists, along with other health and social welfare professionals have found themselves in an ever-expanding demand for their services.

Now, in the twenty-first century, drug misuse poses a major challenge for health professionals and many of the health problems associated with drug misuse can be managed effectively in primary care, utilising the well-established network of primary care professionals. Community pharmacists are ideally placed to become involved in treatment and prevention strategies which may involve collaborative working between a number of professionals ranging from specialist medical and nursing care, through primary care, to support from social services. However, there are several generations of practising community pharmacists who have had little or no under-graduate or postgraduate training in the management of drug misuse. The quality practice of tomorrow will hinge on there being trained and competent practitioners working in a variety of community pharmacy settings and this book aims to provide the reader with a grounding in the historical, research and practical aspects of community pharmacy and drug misuse.

Like many other socio-medical problems, drug misuse can usefully be considered as a chronic relapsing condition. An additional dimension to this is that the patient's behaviour may have negative consequences not only for themselves and their families, but also for the community as a whole. Furthermore, they often find themselves stigmatised by some health professionals as well as by society in general. However, a non-judgemental and non-stigmatising attitude towards this area of healthcare is an essential starting point for quality care. In the 1999 Government clinical guidelines on managing drug misuse, GPs were reminded of their responsibilities with regard to caring for drug misusers through the General Medical Council statement: "It is...unethical for a doctor to withhold treatment for any patient on the basis of a moral judgement that the patient's activities or lifestyles might have contributed to the condition for which treatment is being sought. Unethical behaviour of this kind may raise questions of serious medical misconduct" (Departments of Health, 1999). This could just as well have been written for community pharmacists.

Not all drug misuse results in dependence, nor does it necessarily result in problems for the user. However, it is important to remember that serious consequences can arise from the misuse of any substance (illicit or prescribed). And it is not just injecting which carries risks; these substances do not need to be injected to result in problems such as dependence, poor health, loss of income and the break-up of a relationship. The most serious consequences are likely to result from the use of illicit substances in a manner which is entirely inappropriate (in particular intravenous injecting), but which provides the dependent drug user with the most rapid and cost-effective use of the substance. In the UK, the illicit drug which creates the majority of work for health professionals is heroin, and therefore the reader will find that much of the book focuses on the management of opioid dependence.

This book has a particularly UK focus, with some chapters providing detailed information on UK drug services and UK law as they relate to the provision of these services. Nevertheless, an international readership is likely to find in all the chapters ideas and concepts that translate to their own experience. The book is aimed at all students of pharmacy and pre-registration pharmacists, any community pharmacist working with drug misusers or any pharmacists considering becoming involved, and anyone concerned with developing and managing primary health care services for drug misusers, in particular opiate dependent patients. This book is not a medical textbook on drug misuse, nor is it a textbook of pharmacology. Excellent books already exist which cover these subjects. This book has been written by experienced professionals in the field, and, where possible, uses an evidence-based approach whilst remaining focussed on the practicalities of service provision.

Whilst focussing on drug misuse, in particular the misuse of illicit drugs, two other areas of misuse and dependence also represent huge challenges to health and society – the use of alcohol and tobacco. The impact of brief interventions in primary care in these areas has been shown to be positive. Whilst tobacco and alcohol use are beyond the scope of this book, it is essential to bear in mind that community pharmacists can become involved in prevention and treatment services in this context. Furthermore, those who misuse illicit drugs may also be misusing these substances, further compromising their health.

The reader will note that chapter authors use different terminology to describe issues and individuals. We have left it to the discretion of the individual authors to choose the term they prefer. However, the terms drug misuser, drug user and problem drug user can, in many instances, be used interchangeably, whilst the terms client and patient are used to refer to a person who seeks treatment or a service such as needle exchange. And finally, the terms drug misuse, problem drug use and substance misuse are all used in the book to describe the inappropriate, non-medical use of a drug, sometimes prescribed or obtained through over-the-counter purchase, but more commonly obtained illicitly.

So what is the book about? We have sought answers to a number of questions that have a direct bearing on the development and future of community pharmacy involvement in services for substance misusers.

Our first question was "what is the history of drug misuse in the UK and the history of community pharmacy involvement"? In Chapters 2 and 3, experts in the history of drug misuse and the role of community pharmacy review the historical context in which to consider contemporary development. In Chapter 2, John Witton and colleagues provide us with a review of the UK drug scene from the early part of the twentieth century up to date, detailing some of the major legal and political decisions which have shaped the treatment of drug misuse in the UK today. In Chapter 3, Stuart Anderson and Virginia Berridge treat us to a walk through the history of community pharmacy and its relationship with drug misuse, from the early days when pharmacists could sell opium in their pharmacies – through to the tightly regulated and more integrated services of today.

Next, we ask "what can we learn from research carried out in this field"? The four chapters in this section describe the research and practice of community pharmacists in the UK and the rest of the world. These chapters provide the reader with a review of some of the available evidence about pharmacy's role and effectiveness in service provision and how the evidence informs practice development. In Chapter 7, a brief "voyage" around the world flags up some of the similarities and differences in the way in which countries utilise the services of community pharmacists in the management of drug misuse.

From there we move on to the practical business of service provision and ask "what can be achieved and what are the implications for practising pharmacists"? This is by far the largest section of the book, and provides the reader with a review of some of the approaches adopted by pharmacy – for example, needle exchange and supervised consumption of methadone. Other chapters provide ideas on the potential scope of a pharmacist's involvement in the welfare of drug misusers. The remaining chapters focus on some of the practical and ethical dilemmas faced by pharmacists in the provision of such services, mainly in a UK context, but with relevance to overseas readers.

Finally, we ask "how can community pharmacy contribute further to drug misuse services"? For our concluding section, we have commissioned chapters which focus on the development of community pharmacy through training and multiprofessional working, and finally we attempt to look into the crystal ball and discern the future of this essential cog in the vast machinery which seeks to prevent, treat and alleviate some of the suffering associated with substance misuse.

REFERENCE
Departments of Health *et al.* (1999) *Drug Misuse and Dependence: Guidelines on Clinical Management*, The Stationery Office, London.

Opiate addiction and the "British System": looking back on the twentieth century and trying to see its shape in the future

John Witton, Francis Keaney and John Strang

"Among the remedies which it has pleased Almighty God to give to man to relieve his sufferings, none is so universal and so efficacious as opium".

(Thomas Sydenham, 1680)

INTRODUCTION

Looking back from our vantage point in the twenty-first century on the development of the treatment of drug users in the UK, there are a number of striking aspects of the British approach which are distinctive and have fascinated and perplexed commentators at home and abroad. Figures for 1999 indicate that about 30,000 drug misusers presented to treatment services in a six month period. If we go back forty years, Home Office statistics for 1956 reported 333 addicts in the country (currently the total population of patients of a local drug service). As a recent report observed, it is not just the character of the drug problem that changes like the tide ebbing and flowing; it is also that the sea level has risen dramatically. Yet despite this massive increase in drug misuse over the last forty years there have been features of British drug treatment that have endured. It is the features of this core response which have been dubbed the "British Experience" or "British System".

For many, the British approach to treating drug problems has been marked by the singular lack of a system or, until recently, the lack of a central co-ordinated policy. However, what has struck outside observers as being particularly unique to the British approach is the method of prescribing for drug misusers. Any medical practitioner can prescribe the opiate-substitute methadone or virtually any other drug (apart from the three specific drugs – cocaine, heroin and dipipanone). Only doctors with special licences can prescribe cocaine, heroin or dipipanone. In practice, such licences are granted only to doctors who work in NHS drug clinics and this type of prescribing is very modest. All these drugs can be prescribed either orally or intravenously where appropriate. Whilst guidelines on prescribing practices have attempted to establish recommended practice, there is a wide variation in the amounts of methadone that have been prescribed, anything from 5 mg to an extreme of 1000 mg daily. There is also variation in the preparations of methadone that are available – oral mixture, tablets and injectable ampoules – in a way not seen in other countries. Most of the prescribers had received little or no training in substance misuse and often there is a marked contrast between prescribing habits of NHS practitioners and prescribers in the private sector. Journalists and commentators from abroad often compare this approach with what is happening outside the UK. In particular, British prescribing practice is in stark contrast to the United States where drug treatment is highly regulated and where there are limits on dosage of methadone, take-home privileges and programme content. Furthermore, with few exceptions outside the UK, there is no intravenous prescribing and physicians cannot prescribe heroin or cocaine.

Another striking feature of the British approach, when compared to other countries, is that it allows doctors, in their role as prescribers, a much more flexible approach to the needs of the individual patient. It was only after seventy years of treating drug problems that the first prescribing guidelines *The Guidelines of Good Clinical Practice* were published in 1984 by the Department of Health (Medical Working Group on Drug Dependence, 1984). These guidelines have subsequently undergone a number of revisions and updates in the succeeding years and the most recent updated guidelines, called *Drug Misuse and Dependence – Guidelines on Clinical Management* (commonly termed the "Orange Guidelines" for the colour of the publication's cover), were published in April 1999 (UK Department of Health, 1999). This is a much more comprehensive document that targets general practitioners and emphasises the importance of good assessment, urine testing before prescribing, shared-care, supervised ingestion (where available) and training. It should be noted that these guidelines have no defined legal position, except when they describe legal obligations in relation to the prescribing of controlled drugs (CDs), for example. They are not themselves regulations and the prescribing doctor remains largely unfettered.

So how could the absence of a central regulating system have been accepted for so long? This chapter provides a brief account of the circumstances that gave birth to the British approach and how this British system has evolved through periods of stability and points of crisis unimagined by its devisers. Following this account, attention will be turned to the analysis of current practice in the UK which has formed a notable part of the response to the combined problems of drugs and HIV. The latter part of this chapter focuses on new challenges including the hepatitis C problem and the current state of drug treatment. It then concludes with an appraisal of the options before us three years after the issue of the "Orange Guidelines", with regard to steering the British System in today's increasing international context.

THE EMERGENCE OF THE BRITISH SYSTEM
The roots of the medical approach to the problems of opiate addiction in Britain lie in the nineteenth century and Anderson and Berridge have signposted the key events and debates in Chapter 3. In 1926 the Rolleston Committee established the template for the treatment of drug problems for the next forty years and its significance for this chapter is the latitude it accorded to doctors for prescribing to drug dependent patients (UK Ministry of Health, 1926). The report established the right of medical practitioners to prescribe regular supplies of opiates to certain patients which the

Committee regarded as "treatment" rather than "gratification of addiction". This move firmly defined addiction as a medical condition and as a problem for medical treatment. In such situations, prescribing might occur in the following circumstances:

"i) where patients were under treatment by the gradual withdrawal method with a view to cure;

ii) where it has been demonstrated after a prolonged attempt to cure, that the use of the drug could not be safely discontinued entirely on account of the severity of the withdrawal symptoms produced; and

iii) where it has been similarly demonstrated that the patient, while capable of leading a useful and normal life when a certain minimum dose was regularly administered, became incapable of this when the drug was entirely discontinued" (UK Ministry of Health, 1926).

Thus the UK followed a path altogether different from that adopted by the US. In the US, the passage of the Harrison Act in 1914 and subsequent legislation identified drug addiction as a deviant and criminal activity. In contrast in Britain, whilst the possession of dangerous drugs without a prescription was still the subject of the criminal law, opiate addiction became the legitimate domain of medical practice (and hence prescribing) where maintenance doses were allowed (even though this terminology might not have been used). This balance of a medical approach within a penal framework formed the basis of what was to become known as the British System for dealing with drug addiction.

As noted by Anderson and Berridge, calm seems to have prevailed on the British drug scene for the next forty years, and the American commentators at the time and subsequent commentators have eulogised about the effectiveness of the British System of these years – certainly in comparison to the continued and growing problems in the US. Schur identifies a total of 14 key characteristics of this British System including a small number of addicts around which it revolved, the absence of any illicit traffic in drugs, the absence of any addict crime or special subculture, the absence of any young drug users, and a high proportion of addicts from the medical profession and other socially stable circumstances (Schur, 1966). However, other commentators have questioned whether this quiet state of affairs was a result of the success of the system. As Bewley commented, in fact "there was no system, but as there was very little in the way of misuse of drugs this did not matter" (Bewley, 1975).

The Brain Committee and the drug crisis of the 1960s

Up until the 1950s, it was thought that the majority of addicts were of therapeutic origin, and were middle-aged or elderly people who were prescribed opiates in the course of the treatment of illness with a second category being "professional addicts" – doctors, dentists and pharmacists who became addicted partly through their professional access to dangerous drugs. In the early 1950s, the first signs of an American-type opiate problem occurred in London, following a theft of hospital drugs (Spear, 1994). Reports about the activities of young heroin users began to appear in the British newspapers such as had not seen before in the UK. Claims were made that drug sub-cultures were forming, mainly in London. These events prompted the two Brain Committee reports.

The key question the second Brain Committee addressed was whether these changes in the patterns and extent of drug use required a new approach. In their evidence, the second Brain Committee learned that the increased use of opiates related in particular to heroin for which the annual total number of addicts known to the Home Office had risen from 68 to 342 in the preceding five years, and was accompanied by a similar increase in the number of known cocaine addicts from 30 to 211 in the same period. Virtually all of these were combined heroin and cocaine addicts. These new addicts were predominantly young males living in the London area. The Committee soon established that there was no evidence of any black market imported heroin, and expressed their concern about the over-generous prescribing of such drugs, observing that "supplies on such a scale can easily provide a surplus that will attract new recruits to the rank of addict".

A rethinking of policy was urgently required as the pre-existing British System was clearly failing to limit the spread of youthful heroin addiction and actually appeared to be contributing to the spread of the problem by making supplies so easily available. Drug addiction was reformulated as a socially infectious condition for which it was appropriate to provide treatment. The second Brain Committee believed that control of the drug problem could be exercised only through control of the treatment. Three linked proposals formed the basis of the second Brain Report: restriction on the availability of heroin, the introduction of special drug treatment centres and the introduction of the notification system for addiction (as with infectious diseases).

The arrival of the specialist clinics

As a result of the Brain Committee's recommendations, special drug clinics were established in the spring of 1968, to coincide with the introduction of the new Dangerous Drugs Act (1967). Prescribing restrictions were introduced and only specially licensed doctors could prescribe heroin and cocaine to addicts. The aim was to exclude the naive or corrupt prescribing doctor, for, as Connell said at the time "all professional classes contain weaker brethren" (Connell, 1969). The brief for these new clinics had been outlined in the recommendations from the Ministry of Health which identified that, in addition to providing appropriate treatment to drug addicts, the aim was also to contain the spread of heroin addiction by continuing to supply this drug in minimum quantities where it was necessary, depending on the doctor, and where possible to persuade addicts to accept withdrawal treatment. As Stimson and Oppenheimer subsequently commented, new clinics were given the twin briefs of medical care and social control.

The early years of the clinics

By 1968 there were approximately 60 doctors licensed to prescribe heroin and cocaine, with 39 clinics providing treatment, 15 in London and 24 in other parts of England and Wales. Practitioners treating drug users were obliged to notify the Home Office of their cases for inclusion on the Addicts Index and 1,306 addicts were notified in 1968, the first year of operation of both the new clinics and the Addicts Index. Most of them were dependent on heroin and living in the London area. The clinics established in the London area saw 79% of the notified opiate addicts in England and Wales in 1968. Frequently the doctor working at the clinic would initially prescribe heroin and/or cocaine at doses similar to those previously prescribed by the private doctor. Thereafter the average daily dose of prescribed heroin fell steadily over the next few years and there was a gradual establishment of injectable methadone and then subsequently oral methadone as a substitute for opiate drugs, which might be prescribed in combination with heroin. Cocaine was initially prescribed in an injectable form at the drug clinics, but this almost entirely ceased in late 1968 following a voluntary agreement between clinic doctors.

The methylamphetamine epidemic
During 1968, a new major problem emerged – the abuse of intravenous amphetamines. One particular private doctor had begun to prescribe methylamphetamine ampoules to drug addicts and widespread use of this drug in the London area followed. A short lived experiment into the possible value of prescribing injectable amphetamines to these patients in order to stabilise their lifestyles and eventually weaning them off, was largely a record of therapeutic failure. By the end of 1968 voluntary agreement had been reached between the Department of Health, the Drug Clinics and the manufacturers of the methylamphetamine ampoules, so that the drug was withdrawn from supply to retail pharmacies. Thereafter the drug was, in effect, available only through the drug clinics, which chose not to prescribe. This attempt to manipulate drug availability to stunt this emerging epidemic appeared to be successful.

The clinics in the middle years
After the initial impact of the introduction of the new drug clinics, there came the gradual realisation of the cumulative enormity of the problem being tackled. Although the clinics had some success in attracting addicts to their services even before the early years, evidence had emerged that pointed to the existence of a large population of drug addicts who remained out of contact with them. Many of these patients had been taken on with actual or presumed promises of life-long maintenance on injectable drugs. The optimistic original view had been that frequent contact between clinic staff and the patient would inspire the demoralised addict to undergo withdrawal. However, all too often, the change within the psychotherapeutic relationship was in the opposite direction, with the secure supply of pharmaceutical injectable drugs legitimately provided by the clinics, entrenching the addict in his/her drug taking ways as institutionalisation set in.

By the mid 1970s, London drug clinics appear to have undergone a collective existential crisis with regard to whether their prime responsibility was for care or for control. Rules were introduced to limit the distracting impact of some behaviours. Fixing rooms in which the addict and fellow users could inject their drugs gradually disappeared from the drug clinics and from the non-statutory agencies. A more active and confrontational style of working became more common in the practice of the clinics. No doubt this was partly born out of contact with the new drug therapeutic community such as Phoenix House, and partly out of a sense of stagnation resulting from the profound lack of personal progress, for many of the maintenance patients. There was an active discussion as to the relative merits of the three main drugs of prescribing, injectable heroin, injectable methadone and oral methadone. A study was conducted at one of the London drug clinics where 96 confirmed heroin addicts were randomly assigned to either injectable heroin or oral methadone maintenance and were followed up for a one year period. The investigators concluded "prescribing injectable heroin could be seen as maintaining the status quo, with the majority continuing to inject heroin regularly to supplement their maintenance prescription from other sources"; whilst refusal to prescribe heroin and offering oral methadone "... resulted in a higher abstinence rate, but also a greater dependence on the illegal source of drugs for those who continued to inject" (Hartnoll *et al.*, 1980). The authors drew attention to these mixed conclusions which did not suggest the superiority of one approach over the other, but that the approach adopted depended on the aims of the service: whether to maximise the numbers who achieve abstinence or to "maintain greater surveillance over a higher number of drug users and ameliorate their total pre-occupation with illicit drug use and criminal activity".

Stimson and Oppenheimer identified three arguments put forward by clinic staff as a need to change direction. Firstly, the legal prescription of opiates had not and never could entirely abolish a large-scale black market in opiates, let alone another drug. Secondly, control of drug use was not an appropriate role for treatment agencies and should be left to legislators and law enforcers. Thirdly, there were practical problems associated with maintaining addicts on injectable drugs when they eventually started running out of veins (Stimson and Oppenheimer, 1992). It is important to realise that there was no central absolute direction to the operation of drug clinics. As a leading consultant said "each physician in charge of a special drug dependence area is a law unto himself, as to how he treats and manages patients".

Consequently clinics began to introduce a policy that only oral methadone could be available for new patients, and by the end of the 1970s, most of the drug clinics had followed this pattern. Thus by the end of the decade a strange situation pertained involving a therapeutic apartheid between those patients who had attended early on (who often still retained maintenance supply of injectable drugs) and those who were taken on by the clinics at a later date (who were offered only oral methadone). The combined shift of prescribing policy and introduction of therapeutic contracts gave the clinic staff a new sense of purpose and direction, with their energies directed toward helping the drug user to be abstinent.

THE BRITISH SYSTEM IN THE EIGHTIES: NEW EPIDEMICS AND NEW POLITICS

The eighties brought new pressures on the treatment system. Already struggling with the care or control contradictions of the previous decade the clinics now had to deal with a new epidemic of heroin use generated by the opening of new trade routes for black market heroin from Iran, Afghanistan, Pakistan and other parts of the "Golden Crescent". The number of addicts notified to the Home Office rose to over 12,000 in 1988, more than twice the number recorded three years before. The amount of heroin seized by customs had increased dramatically and the price of heroin had fallen by 20% between 1980 and 1983. The new wave of heroin addiction occurred particularly in the run-down inner city areas devastated by the restructuring of the British economy in the early 1980s (Pearson, 1987). Unemployed and with no future insight these new young heroin users favoured inhaling heroin, "chasing the dragon", in the mistaken belief that it was not addictive. This belief may have contributed to the increased popularity of the drug and consequently the ever growing number of new heroin users. However, preferred patterns and routes of use were still very localised with injecting still popular in areas like Edinburgh in contrast to the new "chasers" in the northwest of England while heroin users in London favoured both injecting and smoking.

Widespread media coverage made this new wave of heroin use impossible to be ignored and drug use became an important and sustained policy issue for politicians for the first time since the sixties. The Conservative government of the day sought to encourage a coordinated response from across the range of governmental departments through the setting up of an interdepartmental working group of ministers and officials. Significantly the chair of this group was a Home Office minister and when the first government strategy document *Tackling Drug Misuse* was issued in 1986, three of the strategy's five main aspects were enforcement-related and with the health care elements looking like an imposed afterthought. This was probably an accurate reflection of the political view and hence represented a further decline in the primary nature of a medical response to drug problems.

New directions for treatment and an expansion of services

Against this backdrop in 1982 new ways of working within the British System were developed following the recommendations of the *Treatment and Rehabilitation* report from the Advisory Council on the Misuse of Drugs (ACMD). This report signalled a move away from an exclusive reliance on medically-led specialist treatment. The report had three main guiding principles. Following developments in the alcohol field the focus of treatment became the "problem drug user". Drug takers were now recognised as a heterogeneous group with a myriad of problems beyond the use of the drug itself, encompassing social and economic as well as medical problems. The generalist was brought back into the fold as a key to dealing with drug-related problems and drug use was no longer seen as the sole province of the specialist clinic psychiatrist. Finally the local nature of drug problems was recognised by the introduction of Community Drug Teams in towns, cities and counties across the country. These CDTs were based in each health authority and were to provide most of the services formerly provided by the DDUs. Whilst expected to be able to deal with most of the demand for treatment, they had recourse to Regional Drug Problem Teams for expert advice on how to deal with the more difficult cases. In a move to recognise the multidisciplinary impact of drug use, each district health authority would have a District Drugs Advisory Committee and each regional health authority a Regional Drugs Advisory Committee. These advisory committees would have representatives from the gamut of helping agencies including the CDTs, voluntary agencies, general practitioners, probation and social services. Although medical practitioners were still to take the leading role, the emphasis was now on multidisciplinary working.

Guidelines for doctors

In order to encourage the generalist to take a more active role in the treatment of drug use, the Department of Health convened a Medical Working Group on Drug Dependence which produced *Guidelines of Good Clinical Practice in the Treatment of Drug Misuse* which were issued to all doctors in 1984. The guidelines underwent further revision and expansion in succeeding years (1991, 1994 and 1999). Its main themes were to encourage the GP to help any drug using patients through more straightforward approaches like methadone withdrawal, but to look to the specialist drug misuse services for help where longer term prescribing of opioids seemed indicated.

These guidelines were seen by some as an encroachment on the independence of those seeking to treat heroin users and the private prescribing doctor re-emerged to take part in the wider treatment debate. These private doctors saw themselves as providing a service to those who were not ready for the abstinence goal set by the clinics, whilst the clinic specialists viewed the prescribing regimes of these doctors as counter-productive and inimical to the acceptable prescribing policies forged in the preceding decade. The debate continues, with a recent Home Office consultation document seeking to reinforce the standards set out in the most recent clinical guidelines by proposing to extend licensing to doctors who treat drug users with CDs other than oral methadone. As the Department of Health is allocating £3.4 million for the training of all levels of doctors on drug misuse, the role of the prescribing GP is likely to be a contested area for some time to come.

The Central Funding Initiative

These developments were underlined by central government in the form of finance specifically directed at funding drug services in the Central Funding Initiative of 1983. This funding led to a dramatic expansion of the drugs field – for both statutory and voluntary agencies. The national initiative aimed to displace the previous London-based specialist hospital system as the core of the drug treatment approach. Between 1983 and 1987, £17.5 million was made available for the development of new community based services, with over 42% of this money being administered by the voluntary sector. Many small voluntary agencies and residential centres providing care for drug users sprang up in the wake of this initiative but their longevity was uncertain due to the pump-priming nature of the grant-giving (MacGregor *et al.*, 1991).

Dealing with AIDS/HIV

As the increase in service provision began to bed down, the mid-eighties saw the emergence of HIV and AIDS as the dominant public health concern. Injecting drug users, through their sharing of contaminated injecting equipment, were seen as a potential route for the HIV virus to rapidly diffuse into the wider community. The first governmental reaction came in the 1986 report from the Scottish Home and Health Department which introduced the concept of 'safer drug use' and proposed making sterile needles and syringes available to those who inject drugs. Improved treatment services and substitute prescribing were also seen as ways of reducing sharing levels and the spread of HIV infection. Through 1986 a small number of drug agencies began distributing syringes and later in the same year a pilot syringe exchange scheme was set up in England and Scotland. In response to this widespread concern the ACMD set up an AIDS and Drug Misuse Working Group. The subsequent report *AIDS and Drug Misuse Part I* provided the template and rationale for a reorientation of drug treatment practice to meet the new challenge of drugs/HIV. The report stated that "The spread of HIV is a greater threat to individual and public health than drug misuse. Accordingly, we believe that services which aim to minimise HIV risk behaviour by all available means should take precedence in development plans" (Advisory Council on the Misuse of Drugs, 1988). Whilst reiterating that prescribing to drug users should still have an identified goal, the report advocated a hierarchy of treating goals whose appropriateness depended on the user. The key aims were to attract seropositive drug misusers into treatment where they could be encouraged to stop using injecting equipment and move away from injecting towards oral use. Decreasing drug use and abstinence were further levels in the hierarchy and so harm minimisation was the core of the policy and received active support from the Government. This report and its sister report *AIDS and Drug Misuse Part II* continued the policy aim of embracing general practitioners and general psychiatrists and involving them more actively in the direct provision of services to address the more general health care needs of drug users, whilst the specialist clinics maintained responsibility for the more complicated needs of the more difficult drug users.

Harm minimisation

This was the period when harm minimisation became a legitimate objective as well as representing a banner under which an increasing number of clinicians and agencies re-focused their energies and work. Harm minimisation, acknowledged as the crucial approach to drug use was characterised by adopting measures that sought to reduce the harm caused by continued drug use and to seek a modification of the continued use of drugs. This approach recognised that many injecting drug users were unwilling or unable to stop injecting and that advice on how to clean needles and syringes would often be unheeded by users. Up to this time clean needles and syringes were difficult to obtain in many parts of the country and pharmacists were often unwilling to knowingly sell needles and syringes to drug users. A consequence of this situation became apparent in Edinburgh when within only a few years of the first case of HIV in the city, around half of the city's heroin users were found to be already infected with the virus. The introduction of needle exchange schemes were a reflection of this changed "harm minimisation" approach. Voluntary and health service agencies led the way in establishing centres where injecting drug users were able to obtain sterile injecting equipment.

The re-emergence of maintenance

In the light of the new public health reappraisal, maintenance prescribing once again moved centre stage – on this occasion in the form of oral methadone maintenance. Over the previous couple of decades, an impressive body of evidence in support of oral methadone maintenance had been established (especially from the US) which demonstrated its effectiveness at promoting, among other benefits, marked reductions in continued heroin use and continued injecting. In the new climate these particular benefits are obviously much sought after and the publication and wider presentation of reviews of this evidence (Ward *et al.*, 1992; Farrell *et al.*, 1994) contributed to the wider acceptance in the UK of oral methadone maintenance as a central plank of the combined drug/HIV treatment response.

1990s: CRIME REDUCTION TO THE FORE

By the early 1990s, it had become clear that the UK had not seen the major spread of HIV infection among injecting drug users that many had feared. However, the "drug problem" remained high on the wider political agenda and new policy developments continued. With the growth of recreational drug use in the late 1980s and early 1990s and the increasing acceptability of drug use amongst adolescents and young adults the government published *Tackling Drugs Together: a strategy for England 1995–1998*. It sought to combine "accessible treatment" with "vigorous law enforcement . . . and a new emphasis on education and prevention". The aim of the strategy was to increase community safety from crime and to reduce the health risks and other damage related to drug use. A Department of Health Task Force was established to examine the effectiveness of treatment in order to help health purchasers decide what kind of treatment was needed and how it should be given. The Task Force had been set up in 1994 and surveyed current practice and cost-effectiveness of treatment services and examined current treatment policy. It commissioned new research to generate evidence including the National Treatment Outcomes Research Study. This study recruited a sample of 1000 drug users from four types of treatment modality, methadone maintenance, methadone reduction, residential rehabilitation programmes and specialist drug dependence units and intended to follow their progress over five years.

Among the widely-publicised findings from NTORS (National Treatment Outcome Research Study) was the observation that treatment was associated with major reductions in criminal behaviour (Gossop *et al.*, 1998a,b) – to such an extent that it was possible to calculate that each pound spent on treatment was associated with three pounds reduction in the costs to society (largely as a result of reduced levels of acquisitive crime and associated costs of the criminal justice system). This finding became public at a time when the drug–crime link was already becoming the dominant political concern about drug misuse (having overtaken HIV and health concerns as the main driving force), and hence resulted in a strange strategic alliance between law enforcement and the call for greater access to treatment.

A further strategy document followed in 1998, building on the themes of its predecessor and emphasising collaboration and partnership between different agencies. Amongst the aims of *Tackling Drugs to Build a Better Britain: the Government's Ten-Year Strategy for Tackling Drug Misuse* was to help people with drug problems to overcome them and live crime-free lives. The report was preceded by the appointment, for the first time in the UK, of an Anti-Drugs Coordinator (drug "czar") in January of that year. In the Coordinator's first annual report, performance indicators were provided, to support the strategy which included increasing the numbers in treatment to 66% by 2005 and to 100% by 2008. An extra £20.5 million for social services and £50 million for health authorities was expected to increase the treatment numbers by a third.

Treatment was thus re-conceptualised as an intervention which might lead to reduction of criminal behaviour. Drug using criminals were encouraged to enter treatment as a means of altering their behaviour. Policy initiatives and resources were introduced to link the criminal justice system and the treatment sector through DTTOs (Drug Treatment and Testing Orders). Under the Criminal Justice and Court Services Bill, drug testing of offenders could be introduced at every stage of the criminal process with an aim of identifying those offenders who should be getting treatment. The initial findings from NTORS were taken as proof that treatment "worked" in terms of reducing the criminality of drug users and was taken to provide a research rationale for the intermeshing of criminal justice and treatment aims.

More recent developments have reflected this trend. The 2000 Spending Review secured additional funding for the expansion of drug treatment services. As a consequence, Drug Action Teams are now required to complete treatment plans for ratification by the drug strategy coordinating body, the United Kingdom Anti-Drug Coordinating Unit (UKADCU). In drawing up these plans, the involvement of the statutory partners – Health, Local Authorities, Police and Probation – is seen as essential. A National Treatment Agency (NTA) has been set up to ensure coordination of treatment services and set minimum standards for drug treatment under the auspices of the Department of Health, the Home Office and the Anti-Drugs Coordination Unit. The Agency was established as a special health authority to give it "operational independence... in order to become the authoritative national voice on setting standards for drug treatment, commissioning and provision" (UK Department of Health *et al.*, 2001). It is responsible for ensuring equity of access to treatment; addressing the needs of currently under-represented groups; ensuring consistency with other parts of the drug strategy and ensuring effective transitions between different treatment settings such as prison and the community. It was clear that treatment services are seen as crucial to the success of the drug strategy and this was recognised by the doubling of central drug allocation for drug treatment from £63 million in 2000–2001 to £120 million by 2003–2004. But with recent estimates suggesting that criminal justice drug treatment referrals are expected to increase demand by 33% by 2002, it remains to be seen whether the increased investment is enough to support drug treatment services in meeting these raised expectations.

CONCLUSION: HAS THE BRITISH APPROACH HAD ITS DAY?

Do these recent developments mean a further erosion of the British System, with criminal justice and community safety concerns over drug-related crime overwhelming the health rationale of treatment or is it a further realignment between treatment and other policy objectives? The first 80 years of the British System has demonstrated the flexibility of the British approach and its ability to adapt itself to meet new challenges and policy demands – to help limit the impact of the illicit drug market in the 1960s and 1970s through to the reduction of the spread of HIV and AIDS in the 1990s. Many of the fundamental conflicts about the purpose of treatment and prescribing practice still are unresolved while tighter guidelines and the demands for higher treatment standards throughout the health field further circumscribe the prescribing doctor's freedom of manoeuvre. Recent concerns about the spread of hepatitis C among injecting drug users demonstrate that serious health risks associated with drug use are always emerging which treatment practice has to evolve to deal with, and new treatment practices will continue to be essential as part of the coordinated response. While society's opinions on the weightings that has to be attached to different outcomes will vary over time, it remains the case, for the foreseeable future, that several of the existing treatments have such a solid research foundation that they will continue to be seen as essential evidence-based practice in the 'British System' of the future. However, it remains less clear, at the time of writing, whether the driving force for this treatment expansion will continue to be society's concern about the health and well-being of an young addicted population or whether the treatment provision will be primarily in response to concerns about public safety and the escalating costs of drug-related crime.

REFERENCES

Advisory Council on the Misuse of Drugs (1988). *AIDS and Drug Misuse, Part 1*, HMSO, London.

Bewley TH (1975). Evaluation of addiction treatment in England. In: Bostrom H, Larsson T, Ljungstedt N. (eds) *Drug Dependence: Treatment and Treatment Evaluation*, Almqvist & Wiksell, Stockholm, pp. 275–286.

Connell PH (1969). Drug dependence in Great Britain: a challenge to the practice of medicine. In Steinberg H. (ed) *Scientific Basis of Drug Dependence*, Churchill, London.

Edwards G (1969). The British approach to the treatment of heroin addiction. *Lancet*, I, 768–772.

Farrell M, Ward J, Des Jarlais DC, Gossop M, Stimson GV, Hall W, Mattick R, Strang J (1994). Methadone maintenance programmes: review of new data with special reference to impact on HIV transmission. *British Medical Journal*, 309, 997–1001.

Gossop M, Marsden J, Stewart D, Lehmann P, Edwards C, Wilson A, Segar G (1998a). Substance use, health and social problems of service users at 54 drug treatment agencies. *British Journal of Psychiatry*, 173, 166–171.

Gossop M, Marsden J, Stewart D (1998b). *NTORS at One Year: Changes in Substance Use, Health and Criminal Behaviour One Year After Intake*, Department of Health, London.

Hartnoll RL, Mitcheson MC, Battersby A, Brown G, Ellis M, Fleming P, Headley N (1980). Evaluation of heroin maintenance in controlled trial. *Archives of General Psychiatry*, 37, 877–884.

MacGregor S, Ettore B, Coomber R, Crosier A, Lodge H (1991). *Drug Services in England and the Impact of the Central Funding Initiative*, ISDD, London.

Medical Working Group on Drug Dependence (1984). *Guidelines of Good Clinical Practice in the Treatment of Drug Misuse*, Department of Health and Social Security, London.

Pearson G (1987). *The New Heroin Users*, Blackwell, London.

Schur EM (1966). *Narcotic Addiction in Britain and America: the impact of public policy.* Associated Book Publishers, London.

Spear B (1994). The early years of the 'British System' in practice. In Strang J and Gossop M (eds). *Heroin Addiction and Drug Policy: The British System*, Oxford University Press, Oxford.

Stimson GV, Oppenheimer E (1992). *Heroin Addiction: treatment and control in Britain*, Tavistock, London.

UK Department of Health, United Kingdom Anti-Drugs Co-ordinating Unit, UK. Home Office (2001). *The National Treatment Agency for Substance Misuse: a Consultation Document*, Department of Health, London.

UK Department of Health (1999). *Drug Misuse and Dependence: Guidelines on Clinical Management*, HMSO, London.

UK Ministry of Health (1926). *Report of the Departmental Committee on Morphine and Heroin Addiction (Rolleston Report)*, HMSO, London.

Ward J, Darke S, Hall W, Mattick R (1992). Methadone maintenance and the human immuno-deficiency virus: current issues in treatment and research. *British Journal of Addiction*, 87, 447–454.

3

Drug misuse and the community pharmacist: a historical overview

Stuart Anderson and Virginia Berridge

INTRODUCTION

Today, community pharmacists have an important role in relation to drug misuse. But how did pharmacists come to be involved with dangerous substances? As some substances came to be regarded as "drugs of abuse", and their use came to be defined as a "problem", how did the role of community pharmacists in the control of such drugs change as policy unfolded? These are the key historical questions we aim to address in this chapter.

In Great Britain, in the nineteenth century limited control over a number of substances, including opiates, was implemented through the emergent pharmaceutical profession. However, the initial primacy of pharmaceutical regulation became eclipsed as medical and legal systems vied for supremacy early in the twentieth century. A medico-legal system continued to prevail well into the 1960s. Only recently has the role of the community pharmacist in relation to these drugs again become significant.

In this chapter, we trace the evolution of the pharmaceutical regulation of harmful substances by exploring three main time frames: the rise of the system of pharmaceutical control in the middle of the nineteenth century, following the professionalisation of pharmacy; its marginalisation following passage of the 1920 Dangerous Drugs Act, continuing over the next half century; and the subsequent re-emergence of pharmaceutical regulation from 1980 onwards. We explore this evolution by identifying and describing the key events, or watersheds, which had occurred during this period.

THE RISE OF PHARMACEUTICAL REGULATION 1851–1912

The early period, which saw the rise of the system of pharmaceutical regulation, was underpinned by legislation, most notably the Arsenic Act of 1851, the Pharmacy and Poisons Act of 1868, and later the Poisons and Pharmacy Act of 1908. In this section we consider the background to these developments, and explore their consequences for community pharmacy.

The origins of substance regulation: the Arsenic Act 1851
At the time the Pharmaceutical Society of Great Britain was founded in 1841, there was no control of any kind over any substance, no matter how lethal. Any person could obtain any quantity of even the most toxic material without constraint. There was no substance restricted to prescription by doctors, no need to ask questions about the intended use of poisons or to keep records of their sales, and certainly no penalties for inappropriate supply. The quality of what was supplied was frequently suspect, either through adulteration, inappropriate storage, or defects in preparation (Holloway, 1991).

The consequence of unconstrained supply, ready availability and low cost was unlimited use. Poisonous substances were used in large quantities for a wide range of domestic uses. Arsenic and strychnine were supplied in huge quantities for a wide range of agricultural and other purposes. Other potent substances were liberally used in the preparation of medicines. There were no labelling requirements. Usually there was no way of knowing what a particular medicine contained. It might have contained a potent substance, or it might have only been a little more than a flavoured water.

In the late 1840s public concern first emerged about the unrestricted availability of poisons. Reports from the Registrar General's Office, which had been established in 1837, began to draw attention to the large number of deaths resulting each year due to poisoning. More than one third of these resulted from the use of arsenic. In 1849, several cases of murder by arsenic poisoning were reported in the newspapers, and there was a widespread perception of an outbreak of secret poisoning, with chemists and druggists branded as traffickers. Many solutions to the problem were proposed, including a total ban on the retail sale of arsenic, and the reporting of every sale to the nearest police station.

A number of institutions stepped into this situation. The Provincial Medical and Surgical Association (founded in 1832 and becoming the British Medical Association in 1855) represented the views of the doctors. The Pharmaceutical Society of Great Britain (founded in 1841) represented the chemists and druggists. Both bodies took the opportunity to signal their involvement in this area. In 1849, the Pharmaceutical Society undertook a survey of its members' involvement in the sale of poisons. The results were published in a report that established the Society's credentials as an authority in such sales.

The two professional associations put forward joint proposals to the Home Secretary, and these formed the basis of the Arsenic Act of 1851. For the first time the retail sale of a poison was to be restricted. Records of every sale had to be kept, the purchaser (who must be an adult) must be known to the seller, and the arsenic had to be mixed with soot or indigo (to colour it black or red). Provided these conditions were met, anyone could trade in arsenic: there was no pharmaceutical monopoly. With no adequate provision for enforcement, the Arsenic Act was only a little more than a statement of intent.

Poisons, drugs and medicines: use, abuse and misuse
Up until the middle of the nineteenth century, opium and other drugs were on open sale and in popular use. Opium in one form or another was ubiquitous. It was widely prescribed by doctors for its pain relieving and calming properties. It was contained in a large number of proprietary medicines. Laudanum (opium tincture) was to be found in most homes as an essential standby, for use either on its own or as an

ingredient of a home remedy. It was commonly used as an infant soother, to keep babies quiet, and its deliberate use to effect death, either by suicide or murder, was well known. What would now be termed "addiction" was widespread at the time, but the term had no meaning or social significance in the context of the nineteenth century. Likewise, the distinction that is drawn today between legitimate medical and illegitimate non-medical usage had no meaning at that time, when self-medication with potent substances was common (Berridge, 1999).

Inevitably, significant number of people became dependent on it. But their dependence was not seen as an "illness", or as something that had to be treated by a medical practitioner. Rather it was a condition that could be sustained. Legitimate supplies could be obtained through the usual channel of the chemist, and life could be led more or less normal. The system of pharmaceutical regulation was concerned more with the availability of dangerous substances, than with their use.

The impact of the Arsenic Act on criminal poisoning was minimal. In the late 1850s, a series of cases received a great deal of press coverage, and calls for greater control over the sale of a wide range of poisons followed. Several attempts at legislation were made, initially without success. It was not until May 1868, that a bill produced by the Pharmaceutical Society to regulate the sale of poisons was introduced in the House of Lords. An early draft of the bill had been provided for the regulation of opium, but this had been withdrawn by the Society's Council following lobbying by a group of druggists who believed that its regulation would have a serious impact on their trade.

The regulation of poisons: the Pharmacy and Poisons Act 1868

An attempt to limit the supply of powerful drugs being prescribed by medical practitioners was also defeated. The position of the Pharmaceutical Society was that the most effective safeguard in the supply of poisons to the public was to restrict their sale to pharmaceutical chemists, who would be able to exercise their professional judgement and responsibility. The outcome was the Pharmacy and Poisons Act of 1868, which largely extended arrangements made under the Arsenic Act to a range of twenty commonly used poisons, including opium, strychnine and prussic acid. A pharmaceutical system of regulation had prevailed.

Developments over the decades that followed were to confirm and consolidate this arrangement. Sales of proprietary medicines increased spectacularly with the rise in working class buying power. Sales increased nearly tenfold over the fifty years between 1855 and 1905, whilst the population barely doubled. Medicine licence duty, required for the retail sale of medicines, was reduced in 1875, leading to an increase in the number of vendors from about 13,000 in 1874 to 20,000 in ten years. Some of the proprietary medicines available contained dangerous concentration of powerful drugs, such as morphine, strychnine and aconite. Only a small number were labelled "poison" as required by law, and none actually listed the ingredients on the bottle.

During the 1880s, attempts were made to bring proprietary medicines under professional control. But the doctors, and the chemists and druggists had different objectives. The doctors wanted medicines containing poisons to be available only on prescription, while the chemists and druggists were more concerned with preventing unqualified persons from selling them. Concerns about the number of deaths resulting from chlorodyne, the main ingredients of which were morphine and chloroform, led to a campaign against all proprietary medicines by the *British Medical Journal*.

A number of legal cases led to the sale of all proprietary medicines containing scheduled poisons being restricted to registered chemists. The Pharmaceutical Society vigorously prosecuted any unqualified dealer who attempted to sell them.

The medical backlash: the Poisons and Pharmacy Act 1908
The medical profession viewed with alarm, the rise of pharmaceutical regulation of dangerous substances. Their attempts to restrict the availability of poisons to prescription only had failed. Their campaign against patent medicines, and hence restriction of self-medication, was driven by self-interest. General practitioners resisted attempts by their own College of Physicians to restrict doctors' involvement in retail trading. An amendment to the 1868 Pharmacy and Poisons Act made it possible for registered medical practitioners to also register as chemists and druggists.

In 1869, the Council of the Pharmaceutical Society produced, under pressure from the Privy Council, a set of detailed regulations detailing how its members should keep, compound and dispense poisons. This generated strong opposition from its members. What caused most resentment was that the medical practitioners, with or without retail shops, would be exempted from the regulations. In effect, the protection of the public required chemists and druggists to have regulations imposed on them from above, whilst medical practitioners could be safely left to their own devices. Chemists and druggists around the country demonstrated their opposition to these proposals, and they were eventually withdrawn.

The incident exposed the limitations of the Privy Council's powers, and demonstrated that concerted efforts by the membership could block attempts by the Pharmaceutical Society's Council to impose regulation on it. But with enactment of the Poisons and Pharmacy Act in 1908, the Pharmaceutical Society retained its powers to deem a substance as poison, to decide which compounds should be available for sale by anyone, and who should be allowed to become both authorised and listed sellers of poisons.

The 1908 Poisons and Pharmacy Act gave pharmacists further responsibilities in relation to the control of poisons in the pre 1920 period. The Act insisted that the purchaser of opiates should be known to the seller, and that an entry should be made in the Poisons Register. But this legislation placed no control over the manufacture or possession of narcotics. Both opium and cocaine were freely available in unregulated quantities without prescription. The Pharmaceutical Society had the task of policing the Act under the general supervision of the Privy Council Office.

Until enactment of the Dangerous Drugs Act in 1920, the only protection against the abuse of these medicines was the professional discretion of the chemist. Such control was largely ineffective. A conscientious chemist might limit sales to one bottle per customer, but the customer was always free to obtain further supplies elsewhere. The medical campaign against patent medicines continued, with articles attacking the "widespread system of home-drugging" which resulted from the ready availability of opiates in proprietary medicines (Anderson and Berridge, 2000a).

In 1909 and 1912, the British Medical Association published *Secret Remedies* and *More Secret Remedies* respectively to educate the public about the true nature of proprietary medicines. After 1900, manufacturers whose remedies once contained opium began to drop it from their formulae. *Liquifruta medica* was guaranteed to be "free of poison, laudanum, copper solution, cocaine, morphia, chloral, calomel,

Table 3.1 Narcotic deaths 1863–1910

Year	Total Narcotic deaths		Accidental Narcotic deaths		Narcotic suicides	
	No.	Per million population	No.	Per million population	No.	Per million population
1863	126	6.1	106	5.1	19	0.9
1864	134	6.4	102	4.9	28	1.3
1865	120	5.7	98	4.6	22	1.0
1866	114	5.3	92	4.3	18	0.8
1867	138	6.4	110	5.1	28	1.3
1868	140	6.4	104	4.7	35	1.6
1869	100	4.5	83	3.7	17	0.8
1870	90	4.0	62	2.8	27	1.2
1871	97	4.3	86	3.8	11	0.5
1872	102	4.4	81	3.5	21	0.9
1873	108	4.6	66	2.8	42	1.8
1874	103	4.3	77	3.2	25	1.1
1875	116	4.8	80	3.3	36	1.5
1876	111	4.6	81	3.3	30	1.2
1877	110	4.5	78	3.2	32	1.3
1878	130	5.2	94	3.8	35	1.4
1879	144	5.7	100	3.9	43	1.7
1880	131	5.1	95	3.7	36	1.4
1881	144	5.5	105	4.0	40	1.5
1882	128	4.9	96	3.6	32	1.2
1883	136	5.1	103	3.9	32	1.2
1884	120	4.5	73	2.7	47	1.7
1885	162	6.0	107	3.9	53	1.9
1886	137	5.0	93	3.4	42	1.5
1887	156	5.6	104	3.7	52	1.9
1888	177	6.3	108	3.8	65	2.3
1889	149	5.2	99	3.5	48	1.7
1890	164	5.7	97	3.4	65	2.3
1891	173	5.9	116	4.0	56	1.9
1892	163	5.5	104	3.5	59	2.0
1893	174	5.8	107	3.6	67	2.3
1894	196	6.5	111	3.7	85	2.8
1895	193	6.3	119	3.9	74	2.4
1896	177	5.7	110	3.6	67	2.2
1897	206	6.6	139	4.5	64	2.1
1898	159	5.0	97	3.1	62	2.0
1899	169	5.3	95	3.0	74	2.3
1900	169	5.2	95	2.9	72	2.2
1901	138	4.2	75	2.3	62	1.9
1902	151	4.6	88	2.7	63	1.9
1903	164	4.9	102	3.1	61	1.8
1904	162	4.8	81	2.4	80	2.4
1905	162	4.8	67	2.0	92	2.7
1906	152	4.4	83	2.4	64	1.9
1907	148	4.3	80	2.3	67	1.9
1908	129	3.7	61	1.7	66	1.9
1909	119	3.4	66	1.9	51	1.4
1910	101	2.8	57	1.6	44	1.2

Source: Registrar General's Reports: Violent Deaths 1863–1911.

paregoric, narcotics or preservative". The system of pharmaceutical regulation began to be reinforced by informed consumer choice.

This pharmaceutical system of regulation had considerable success, and contributed substantially to reduced rates of accidental over-dosage. Deaths from narcotic over-dosage more than halved, from a peak of 206 in 1897, to 101 in 1910. Narcotic suicides declined from 92 in 1905 to 44 in 1910. The numbers of narcotic deaths in England and Wales between 1863 and 1910 are shown in Table 3.1.

There were, of course, other factors contributing to these reductions. Better control of food and drugs resulted in less adulteration. The use of opiates and other addictive substances was declining as a result of other changes in society. The trends were encouraging, and this system of pharmaceutical control may well have continued but for the First World War.

THE MARGINALISATION OF PHARMACEUTICAL REGULATION 1912–1961
The second time frame is characterised by the marginalisation of pharmaceutical regulation, largely resulting from international developments, and lasting for nearly fifty years. Key milestones were the Opium Convention of 1912, and passage of the first Dangerous Drugs Act in 1920.

International developments: the Opium Convention 1912
It was international developments that eventually led to radical change in the system of control of addictive substances. At the instigation of the United States government, a series of conferences was held, beginning at Shanghai in 1909 and culminating in the International Opium Convention which was signed at "The Hague" on 23 January 1912. This committed the signatories to restricting the trade and consumption of drugs to "medical and legitimate uses", and to apply the necessary regulations to all preparations which contained more than 0.2% of morphine or more than 0.1% of either heroin or cocaine.

The initial focus had been opiate use in the Far East. The remit gradually widened, largely to accommodate British and German demands to control morphine and cocaine. A world-wide system of control would require changes in the system of domestic regulation. Pre-war discussions among British civil servants considered the different forms that control might take. All presupposed the continuation of a system of pharmaceutical regulation to meet the Hague requirements.

The origin of prescription only drugs: the Defence of the Realm Act 1916
Throughout the nineteenth century, it was the Privy Council Office (as the central government department of state with overall responsibility for legislation) which had overall responsibility for pharmacy regulation, and the control of medicines and poisons including opiates. The beginning of the First World War brought the Home Office (as the British government department responsible for law and order in England and Wales) which had responsibility for the Inebriates Act, into the key government role in relation to the control of harmful substances. This saw the advent of a harsher system of control. There was, at the time, a great deal of public and press concern about drug use. There was concern about the smuggling of cocaine to India, and of smoking opium and morphine to the Far East and the United States, much of it

transported on British ships via Japan. But in Britain, the key issue was the efficiency of the army, as rumours grew about the rapid spread of the apparently "recreational" use of cocaine among soldiers. Throughout 1915 and early 1916, protests grew about the extent of the opium smuggling.

Domestic regulation was quickly arranged by including it in regulations (number 40B) under the Defence of the Realm Act (DORA), a catch-all Act which served as cover for a wide variety of wartime regulations. An Order made on 11 May 1916 prohibited the sale or supply of cocaine and other drugs to any member of the forces unless ordered by a doctor on a written prescription, dated and signed, and marked "not to be repeated". It was quickly extended to the civilian population by an order-in-council on 28 July 1916. For the first time in Great Britain, a number of drugs became available only with a doctor's prescription. The supremacy of pharmaceutical control had been challenged by a system of medical regulation, and for a few short years this pharmaceutical-medical system prevailed.

The issue of drugs and the army had in fact arisen early in 1916, not because of illicit cocaine sales but through infringements of the Pharmacy Acts by two London stores. In February 1916, Harrods, and Savory and Moore had both been fined for selling morphine and cocaine without complying with the restrictions concerned. The drugs had been sold in the form of gelatine lamels, consisting of small packets of drugs in a handy case, which had been advertised by Savory and Moore in *The Times* as a "useful present for friends at the front". Both firms were prosecuted by the Pharmaceutical Society. Indeed, Sir William Glyn-Jones, the Society's Secretary, acted as prosecuting counsel in the Harrods case, pointing out that "it was an exceedingly dangerous thing for a drug like morphine to be in the hands of men on active service" (Anderson and Berridge, 2000b).

It was in 1916, against this background of both national and international developments, that opium and cocaine became regulated as narcotics rather than as poisons. In Great Britain, the government's proposals for the implementation of The Hague Convention had originally envisaged a prescription proviso only for preparations containing over 1% of morphine, heroin and cocaine. One of the immediate consequences of the Convention was that the morphine content of the official preparation actually increased. The formula for Tincture of Opium (laudanum) which appeared in the British Pharmacopoeia (BP) of 1914 contained the equivalent of one gram of morphine in one hundred millilitres, i.e. a 1% solution. This was stated to be of approximately the same strength as the *Tinctura Opii* of the International Agreement, and is about one-third stronger than the corresponding preparation of the BP 1898. The implication of this was that most supplies of laudanum would remain under pharmaceutical control by means of over the counter sales, rather than under medical control through prescriptions.

The supremacy of legal control: the Dangerous Drugs Act 1920

With the end of the war signatories were obliged to honour their commitment to the Hague Convention under Article 295 of the Treaty of Versailles. It formed the basis of the Dangerous Drugs Act of 1920, which came into force in September of that year. This extended the DORA 40B regulations to a wider range of narcotics, including medicinal opium and morphine. It prohibited the import of opium prepared for smoking, and the import, export and manufacture of raw opium, cocaine, heroin and morphine except under licence. In addition, the manufacture, sale, possession and distribution of preparations containing more than 0.2% of morphine, or more than 0.1% of either cocaine or heroin, was strictly regulated.

The sale of drugs regulated in this way was restricted to medical practitioners and to pharmacists acting on a doctor's written prescription. The sale of narcotic drugs was to be recorded in books open to inspection by the police. Contravention of the Act was to be punishable by a fine of up to £200, or imprisonment for up to six months, or both. There was very little opposition to it, and the Dangerous Drugs Bill passed into law with virtually no controversy. Despite its acceptance by both the medical and pharmaceutical professions, its impact on both of them was to be significant. Passage of the Act marked the beginning of the displacement of a pharmaceutical system of regulation by a medical system of control through the writing of prescriptions, although the full significance of the Act did not become apparent until later in the 1920s.

The rise of medical regulation: the Rolleston Report 1926

The years from 1921 to 1924, saw persistent attempts by the Home Office to impose a completely penal system of control. The rise of such a system led to the marginalisation of both pharmaceutical and medical regulation. Neither profession liked it. The effect of legislation since 1916 has been to limit the use of narcotics to the prescription of a medical practitioner, and to substitute a medically controlled prescription based system for a pharmaceutical system of regulation. Before 1916, there was no requirement for a medical prescription for the supply of opium, whatever the strength; and prescriptions, in any case, remained the property of the patient rather than the prescriber. They could be repeated indefinitely.

This situation only changed with the DORA 40B regulations. This required that a prescription for a dangerous drug should normally be dispensed once only; that where the doctor expressly indicated that it should be repeated it could be repeated not more than twice (i.e. supplied on not more than three occasions); and that in all cases the chemist would retain the prescription after the initial supply, and keep it in a safe place for a period of two years. These requirements were confirmed in the Dangerous Drugs Act of 1920.

There was extensive grass roots opposition in the medical profession to an entirely legal system of control of such substances. It became impossible to exclude the doctors from the system of control and from the formulation of policy. Doctor civil servants within the Ministry of Health took a key role in policy formation. Following protracted discussions between the Home Office and the Ministry of Health, a departmental committee was established to examine the problem, and the Rolleston Report (Sir Humphrey Rolleston was President of the Royal College of Physicians) appeared in 1926. All nine members of the committee were medical men, as was one of its two secretaries. The Report proposed a modified system of control in which doctors would play a key role. It established the disease view of addiction; patients would seek treatment from doctors, who would then use their discretion as to whether or not to prescribe maintenance doses (Berridge, 1980).

In the debates later in the century about the "drug problem" and the "war on drugs", it can be argued that this so-called "British System" prevented Britain from experiencing the worst excesses of the American "war on drugs", which involved criminalisation of both addicts and the doctors who prescribed for them.

It was however, the result rather than the cause of the low number of British addicts, and of the tolerant approach that prevailed over the next forty years. It has been described as "a system of masterly inactivity in the face of a non-existent problem" (Downes, 1988). The principal recommendations of the Rolleston Committee became law through the passage of further Dangerous Drugs Acts. Through these recommendations the doctors had become equal partners: a solely penal system had become a medico-legal one. The medical prescription and the Home Office inspectorate became the primary means of control. The committee symbolized the victory of medical over pharmaceutical systems of control. Pharmacists were relegated largely to being dispensers of prescriptions written by doctors.

The Dangerous Drugs Act is often discussed in isolation from moves to change the regulation of other substances. But it is important to bear in mind that boundaries around what counted as a "medicine" were also being redrawn at the same period. Concern about the regulation of patent medicines has already been referred to. A new category of medicines came into being with the Therapeutic Substances Act of 1925, which is controlled by licence the manufacture, but not the sale or supply, of a range of preparations, the potency or purity of which could not be tested chemically. These included vaccines, sera, toxins and antitoxins.

Essentially, the boundaries between medicinal preparations and "drugs" were being redrawn. The nineteenth-century idea of "the poison", which had legitimated pharmaceutical systems of regulation ("opiates" were regarded as "poisons" rather than as "dangerous drugs") was being replaced. There was to be greater delineation with, on the one hand, more of a role for medical practice in relation to medicinal preparations or "medicines", and more of a role for criminal justice for "drugs" on the other. These boundaries stayed in place until after the Second World War, until further changes took place particularly in the 1960s. The changed definitions in relation to harmful substances meant that the role of the pharmacist was now more indeterminate. In many ways the profession found itself in the middle between the medical system of control and the criminal justice system.

The marginalisation of pharmaceutical regulation: the Pharmacy and Poisons Act 1933

The Home Office did not consider it necessary to consult the Pharmaceutical Society of Great Britain about the Dangerous Drugs Bill of 1920. Although at first disappointed, the Society eventually gave it a cautious welcome after some of its suggestions were incorporated. But when regulations appeared under the Act, the Society's Council took exception to them, since they made an important class of drugs dependent on a doctor's prescription. They sought to reinstate the freedom of the chemist to sell drugs to persons known to them or introduced by a known person. The government was unsympathetic to these grievances, and the Acts of 1923, 1925 and 1932 amended the Dangerous Drugs Act of 1920 in ways that hardly affected the pharmaceutical profession. However, the Pharmacy and Poisons Act of 1933 contained a Fourth Schedule which listed a number of poisons which could only be sold to the public in accordance with a prescription written by a doctor, dentist or veterinary surgeon. These included barbiturates and digitalis preparations. The creation of Schedule Four represented a major increase in the medical profession's control of the supply of drugs to the general public.

But despite the introduction of the medically controlled prescription-based system in 1920, and the creation of Schedule Four to the Pharmacy and Poisons Act of 1933, there remained some leeway for pharmaceutical regulation. The 1920 Dangerous Drugs Act lowered the limits below which products could be supplied without prescription, from 1% to 0.2% of morphine and 0.1% of cocaine and heroin, the levels set at the Hague. The impact of these changes was, not surprisingly, different for over-the-counter medicines than it was for prescription medicines. Manufacturers of patent medicines, for over-the-counter sale, significantly lowered the morphine content of their preparations in order to stay outside the prescription only limit. On the other hand, the quantity of morphine contained in tincture of opium (laudanum), which became available only on prescription, continued at 1%. This strength remained unchanged at the time of publication of the next British Pharmacopoeia, in 1932, and has continued at the same level up to the present time.

The forty year calm: 1920 to 1960
The period between the 1920s and the 1960s has been viewed subsequently as a forty year period of calm. The early years of this period were marked by far greater activity on the international front than at home. Several new treaties were drawn up between 1924 and 1931. The Geneva Convention of 1925 regulated drug distribution, and the Limitation Convention of 1931 limited the manufacture of opiates to the amounts necessary to meet medical and scientific needs. Cannabis was included in the 1925 convention at the request of the Egyptians.

It was, however, a period during which the illicit trade in narcotics changed markedly. At the beginning of the 1920s, organised criminals were involved only at the end of the supply chain. They worked with manufacturers and middlemen to divert legitimately manufactured drugs to consumers. But by the end of the 1930s, they had migrated to the manufacturing end of the chain, owning clandestine drug factories around the world. Drug users who came to the attention of the authorities in Great Britain were few in number and usually of good social standing. They consisted largely of "professional" addicts who were medically connected, and who therefore had access to medical supplies; and "therapeutic" addicts whose addiction had started when narcotics had been used in the treatment of illness. A Home Office drugs branch was first established in 1934, with largely a surveillance and record keeping role.

The legislation that began with the Dangerous Drugs Act of 1920 remained virtually unchanged for over 30 years, until 1951. Following the Second World War a new Act was passed. The Dangerous Drugs Act of 1951 was divided into five parts. Part 1 controlled raw opium, coca leaves, Indian hemp and its resins and preparations; Part 2 prohibited prepared opium, defined as opium prepared for smoking; and Part 3 was concerned with medicinal dangerous drugs, which were those classified as such in the poisons list, including medicinal opium and morphine. However, the limits below which preparations of opium could be sold over the counter remained unchanged.

THE RE-EMERGENCE OF PHARMACEUTICAL REGULATION 1961 TO PRESENT
It was developments in society in the 1960s that led to a re-appraisal of systems of control, and of the re-emergence of some limited pharmaceutical involvement with regard to substance abuse. In this last section we consider the events which led to this outcome.

A review of the system: the First Brain Report 1961

In 1958 the government appointed an Inter-departmental Committee on Drug Addiction to review the arrangements which had been in force since the Rolleston Report of 1926. It was chaired by Dr (later Sir) Russell Brain, and it reported in 1961. The committee concluded that the arrangements which had been put in place thirty years earlier were still appropriate.

But the report was heavily criticised at the time and subsequently for failing to take account of the changes that were taking place in the UK drug scene. At one encounter at a meeting of the Society for the Study of Addiction, the pharmacist at John Bell and Croyden in Wigmore Street, London ("Benny" Benjamin) famously pointed out directly to Dr Brain that the market that he personally knew of was much larger than that discussed in the report.

Reform of the system: the Second Brain Report 1965

The committee was hastily reconvened as a result of two further reports submitted by the Home Office Drugs Inspectorate that confirmed these observations. The Second Brain Report of 1965 proposed maintenance of a modified medical system of control, but introduced several innovations. Somewhat controversially, it proposed compulsory treatment, a proposal which was later dropped. But two key proposals were adopted. Treatment would be provided in specialist psychiatric 'clinics', and there would be a system of notification of addicts. It allowed any doctor to prescribe heroin for medical treatment, thus defusing any opposition to threats to clinical freedom. The Brain Committee also led to the establishment of the Advisory Committee on Drug Dependence in 1967, chaired by Sir Edward Wayne.

The necessary changes were implemented through legislation. The United Nations Single Convention on Narcotic Drugs in 1961 had replaced all earlier international agreements, and following it the United Kingdom introduced the Dangerous Drugs Acts of 1964 and 1965. These controlled the manufacture, import and export of addiction-producing substances and related raw materials. The problem of non-narcotic but habit-forming drugs was addressed by the Drugs (Prevention of Misuse) Act of 1964. The 1967 Dangerous Drugs Act and the 1968 regulations under it governing supply to addicts brought the clinic system into operation.

The legislation was consolidated and extended in the Misuse of Drugs Act of 1971. The Act prohibits all dealings in the drugs listed in its schedules unless specifically allowed. For example, both solid and liquid preparations of medicinal opium containing a maximum strength of 0.2% of morphine are exempt from all restrictions under Regulations made under the Misuse of Drugs Act except that the invoice, or a copy of it, must be kept for two years. Preparations containing more than this amount remain subject to the restrictions of the Misuse of Drugs Regulations 1985. It was also under this Act that a statutory Advisory Council on the Misuse of Drugs was established. The Advisory Council issued its first interim report on rehabilitation and treatment in 1977.

These reconfigurations did not, however, mean the complete abolition of pharmaceutical systems of control. Evidence from formularies and pharmacopoeias indicates that opium based preparations, for example, remained available for use, both for over-the-counter sale (of a range of external products and internal liquid preparations containing 0.2% or less of morphine) and for supply on prescription (of internal liquid preparations containing 0.2% or more of morphine).

Figure 3.1 indicates the total number of official preparations containing opium between the first edition of the British Pharmacopoeia in 1864 and the most recent one in 1998. It illustrates the shift in the official status of opium during this period. From a high of thirty-eight preparations in 1864 the number steadily fell off during the first half of the twentieth century. Between 1914 and 1948 the number of official opium preparations fell from thirty-two to twenty. The number fell below double figures only in 1978, with only a small further loss of preparations occurring during the 1990s. In 1998 a total of seven preparations containing opium remain official in one of the standard references. The British Pharmacopoeia of 1998 includes raw opium, opium tincture, camphorated opium tincture, and concentrated camphorated opium tincture.

THE REDISCOVERY OF THE PHARMACIST: THE EXTENDED ROLE IN THE 1980s

For pharmacists, the impact of the changes of the 1960s and early 1970s was limited. However, by the late 1970s increasing numbers of notified addicts meant that there were more prescriptions to dispense. The impact was felt first by hospital pharmacists. Whilst many patients began to be treated at Drug Dependency Units, others

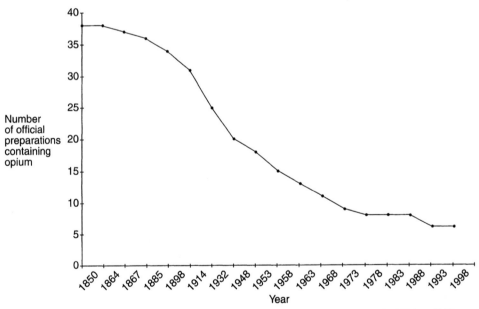

Sources: London Pharmacopoeia 1850; British Pharmacopoeia 1864 to 1998;
British Pharmaceutical Codex 1907–1998; War Formulary 1941–1947;
British National Formulary 1949–1998.

Figure 3.1 Official opium preparations 1850–1998. Reproduced with permission from *Addiction* (2000), 95: 1 (www.tandf.co.uk).

were treated as psychiatric outpatients at hospitals. As a result, increasing numbers of prescriptions for controlled drugs (CDs) were presented at hospital pharmacies. One hospital in Wales experienced a large influx of addicts at the beginning of 1980 due to their inclusion in outpatient clinics (Cherry *et al.*, 1986). Prescriptions for multliples of five milligram units of methadone, as both tablets and linctus, increased from under 2,000 in October 1979 to over 7,000 by October 1980. This was not untypical, and followed the pattern of notifications of addiction to the Home Office during this period. The number of addicts notified to the Home Office between 1971 and 1983 is illustrated in Figure 3.2.

A number of different strategies were implemented to cope with this new development. The closer contact between doctors and pharmacists in hospitals than was normally the case between community pharmacists and general medical practitioners meant that hospital pharmacists often became closely involved in giving product information and prescribing advice to doctors in this area. In southern Derbyshire, for example, a specialist information service on drugs of abuse was established within the Drug Information Centre in 1986. Within a year nearly 5% of all queries at the centre were requests from health professionals for information on drug abuse (Gerrett *et al.*, 1987).

The re-emergence of pharmaceutical involvement was the result of convergence of several factors, principally recognition of a "drug problem", the development of a twin-track policy, and changes in the profession itself. Recognition that there was a "drug problem" was slow in coming. During the 1970s, the reports of the Advisory Committee and the Chief Medical Officer were generally optimistic about it. In Scotland, a specialist subcommittee monitored developments and reported in 1970, 1972, and 1975 (Webster, 1996). The last of these reports expressed "guarded optimism that the problem was diminishing" (Scottish Home and Health Department, 1975).

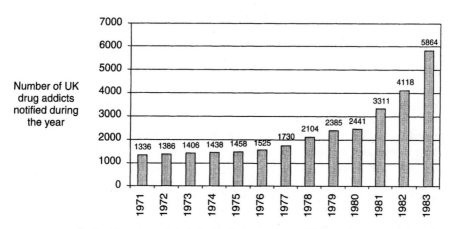

Derived from annual statistical bulletins on drug addicts notified to the Home Office

Figure 3.2 All notifications of opiate and cocaine addicts, United Kingdom 1971–1983.

Drug policy entered a new phase in the early 1980s. The Conservative government took a direct political interest in the drug problem, and advanced a penal response to drugs both nationally and internationally. The 1982 Report on *Treatment and Rehabilitation* by the Advisory Council on the Misuse of Drugs rejected the idea of any pathological or personality defects common to all drug users, and emphasised multi-disciplinary approaches. There should, it stated, be a partnership between the voluntary sector and statutory services, and a new policy community emerged around drugs. This had psychiatric membership, but now embraced a range of interest groups and occupations. There were now two strands to policy: a penal strand driven by the political agenda, and a health strand driven by multi-disciplinary working based on de-medicalisation, community services and harm minimisation.

There was an opportunity here for greater pharmaceutical involvement. Indeed, the re-emergence of pharmaceutical involvement in this area needs to be located in this widening policy community around drugs that became a feature of the 1980s. A broader range of players started to become involved, and the "drug problem" was no longer seen as simply the preserve of psychiatry. Pharmacy's role was probably already set to be part of this change, although it was given a boost by the policy shift that accompanied the arrival of AIDS.

At the same time changes were taking place in the pharmacy profession itself. By the early 1980s there was widespread uncertainty about the future of pharmacy, particularly community pharmacy. The Minister for Health, Dr Gerard Vaughan, announced at the British Pharmaceutical Conference in 1981 that *"one knew there was a future for hospital pharmacists, one knew there was a future for industrial pharmacists, but one was not sure that one knew the future for the general practice pharmacist"* (Anon, 1981).

Pharmacy needed to re-invent itself. Some important initiatives were taken. In 1982, for example, the National Pharmaceutical Association began its "Ask Your Pharmacist" campaign, in which it promoted the use by the public of their local pharmacy. What was really needed, however, was an independent and far-ranging inquiry into the profession. The result was the Nuffield Report. But this comprehensive review of the profession of pharmacy carried out by a committee appointed by the Nuffield Foundation, reporting in 1986, caused pharmacists to examine once again what additional or "extended" roles they might take on (The Nuffield Foundation, 1986).

The tone of the Nuffield report was very positive: "we believe that the pharmacy profession has a distinctive and indispensable contribution to make to health care that is capable of still further development". During the years that followed its publication, pharmacy's leaders were preoccupied with the action necessary to implement the recommendations. Two aspects came to dominate the discussion; whether a pharmacist needed to be on the premises in order to supervise, and the extended role. One such potential extended role was the provision of services to drug misusers. The case for the involvement of community pharmacists in this area was very soon to be reinforced by other developments.

AIDS, DRUG MISUSE AND THE COMMUNITY PHARMACIST

The appearance of AIDS in the early 1980s led most of the health professions to review their roles and priorities. One area where pharmacists were involved was the supply of needles and syringes. This issue clearly illustrated the shifting professional attitudes that characterised this decade. The pharmacy response to the supply of needles and syringes to addicts rapidly moved from disapproval through neutral tolerance to active endorsement in response to external events. Some pharmacists had originally been happy to sell syringes to addicts, but this practice soon came to the attention of their professional body, the Pharmaceutical Society of Great Britain. A Statement by the Council of the Society in 1982 required pharmacists to restrict the sale of syringes and needles "*to bona fide patients for therapeutic purposes*" (RPSGB, 1988a). The intention was that the restriction would be a factor in helping to reduce the increase in the number of drug misusers. This policy was, in fact, in line with official Department of Health policy that saw the supply of needles to addicts as condoning and encouraging heroin misuse. Pharmacy was not to be seen as in any way contributing to a weakening of a punitive drug control policy (Berridge, 1996).

By the mid-1980s there was increasing awareness of the dangers of cross infection, particularly of the HIV virus, involved in parenteral drug abuse. The dangers arose when misusers and registered addicts used and shared contaminated syringes and needles. The fact that pharmacists had been forced by their professional body to stop selling syringes to addicts was the reason given by Dr Roy Robertson, an Edinburgh GP on the Muirhouse estate on the outskirts of the city, whose practice included a large number of addicts, for the spread of the Edinburgh HIV epidemic amongst drug misusers (Robertson, 1990). "Shooting galleries" where twenty or thirty drug users gathered to share one syringe were said to be a major cause of the spread of the virus.

A more "liberal" policy response was called for. Harm minimisation became the key strategy, and the establishment of needle exchange schemes was one strand in it. As with some other health policy initiatives it was Scotland that took the lead. A Scottish Office circular published in June 1988 promoted the sale of syringes through pharmacies. Exchange schemes for syringes and needles had initially been strongly opposed by pharmacists. But eventually, in April 1987, the Council of the Pharmaceutical Society approved guidelines for pharmacists involved in schemes to supply clean syringes and needles to addicts (RPSGB, 1988a). It emphasised that "participation in such schemes is entirely voluntary and at the discretion of the pharmacist involved". After pilot schemes in Liverpool and Bradford the concept of such exchange schemes through pharmacies gradually became more widely accepted by the profession (Blenkinsopp and Panton, 1991).

AIDS therefore provided an opportunity for pharmacists to demonstrate their value in a specific primary care response, by becoming involved in syringe and needle exchange schemes. This was an issue central to the discussion of the developing extended role of the community pharmacist. The history and operation of needle exchange schemes in community pharmacy is discussed more fully in Chapter 9. It is important to note here, however, that work on the role of pharmacists in relation to drug users, including needle exchange schemes, predates the emergence of AIDS.

DRUG MISUSE AND THE EXTENDED ROLE OF THE COMMUNITY PHARMACIST: THE 1990s

The task of considering in what ways the role of community pharmacists might be extended was delegated to a Joint Working Party of the Department of Health and the pharmaceutical profession. This was set up in November 1990 with the following terms of reference; "*to consider ways in which the National Health Service*

Table 3.2 Methadone prescribing: number of methadone hydrochloride prescription items
dispensed in the community by medicament classification, 1991–1999 (England)[a,b]

Description	Prescription items (000s)								
	1991	1992	1993	1994	1995	1996	1997	1998	1999
Injections	39.0	54.5	70.1	81.7	84.2	83.1	85.8	83.1	69.2
Linctuses	6.8	5.3	4.2	4.0	3.5	3.1	2.9	3.0	2.3
Mixtures	403.3	495.0	598.2	682.4	787.0	891.0	981.7	1022.8	1081.7
Others	3.1	4.7	0.2	0.7	1.4	1.0	4.1	3.5	2.8
Tablets	38.3	47.7	62.4	77.3	94.9	97.8	88.8	80.4	69.3
Totals	490.5	607.0	735.1	846.0	970.9	1076.1	1163.2	1192.7	1225.3

Sources: Statistics Division 1E, Prescription Cost Analysis System. London: Department of Health, 1998.

Notes:
a The data cover all prescription items dispensed by community pharmacists and appliance contractors,
  dispensing doctors and prescriptions submitted by prescribing doctors for items personally administered.
b The data cover all prescriptions for methadone hydrochloride and does not identify those solely for drug
  addicts.

*community pharmaceutical services might be developed to increase their contribu-
tion to health care; and to make recommendations"* (RPSGB, 1992).

Its report *"Pharmaceutical Care: the Future for Community Pharmacy"* was
published in March 1992, and it made a total of thirty recommendations. These included
increasing the range of medicines available for sale by pharmacists, the maintenance of
patient medication records by pharmacists, the extension of needle and syringe exchange
schemes, participation in health promotion campaigns, and having separate areas for the
provision of advice and counselling. The recommendations formed the basis for negotiations about the scope of community pharmacy over the years that followed.

The 1990s saw a dramatic increase in the involvement of community pharmacists
in services to drug misusers. A survey of one in every four community pharmacies in
England and Wales indicated that the proportion of respondents dispensing CDs to drug
misusers more than doubled between 1988 and 1995, from 23% to 50%. Methadone
accounted for 96 per cent of such prescriptions in 1995 (Strang et al., 1996). The number
of National Health Service prescriptions for methadone as a drug of dependence dispensed annually in England (excluding hospitals) more than doubled between 1991 and
1999. This is illustrated in Table 3.2.

The proportion of respondents providing a needle exchange service rose from
3–19% during the same period (Sheridan et al., 1996). A similar pattern was seen in
Scotland: the total number of National Health Service prescriptions for methadone
dispensed annually in Scotland (including hospitals) increased from 64,525 in 1992
to 163,833 in 1996 (Pharmacy Practice Division, 1998).

By the mid-1990s community pharmacists throughout Britain were facing
many problems resulting from the large numbers of drug misusers being seen. At
least some of these difficulties were due to constraints imposed by the existing
Misuse of Drugs Regulations, which were seen by many pharmacists as unworkable
in a situation involving such large numbers of prescriptions. The Royal
Pharmaceutical Society of Great Britain increasingly found itself called upon to give

advice to its members. During 1997 two new standards of good pharmaceutical practice were drawn up: standards for pharmacists providing instalment dispensing services were aimed at those involved in the dispensing and supervision of patient self-administration of methadone (as well as other products dispensed on instalment prescriptions); and revised standards for pharmacists providing needle and syringe exchange schemes were produced. Both were accompanied by detailed practice advice (RPSGB, 2000).

By 1997 the Society had concluded that there was an urgent need to review the system for providing services to drug misusers through community pharmacies. It thus established a working group chaired by Mrs Christine Glover, a community pharmacist and Vice-President of the Society. The Report of the Working Party on Pharmaceutical Services for Drug Misusers was published in 1998 (RPSGB, 1998). It made a total of 59 recommendations, the principal one of which was that the government should set up a multi-professional interdepartmental review to produce recommendations for the future management of drug misusers in pharmaceutical primary care.

Together these recommendations represented a shift by the pharmacy profession to a more central and engaged position than it had been in for decades. Pharmacists were responding to changes in the wider society that saw a rise in consumerism and patient empowerment. Drug misusers had been transformed from criminals to service recipients: they were no longer patients but "clients". The working party report had recommended that *"all pharmacists involved in the provision of services to drug misusers should be encouraged, as good practice, to set up patient agreements with their clients where appropriate, in order to safeguard all concerned"*. At least one large chain of pharmacies subsequently introduced a written agreement for drug misuser services for all new clients (Wingfield and Evans, 1999).

Pharmacy's role in this area was soon to gain further support. The Department of Health had set up a Working Party in January 1997 to revise its publication *Drug Misuse and Dependence: Guidelines on Clinical Management*, which had last been revised in 1991. The Group had a broad multidisciplinary membership, which included a pharmacist. In an annex to the report, published in 1999, the roles of a range of health professionals were spelled out (Departments of Health, 1999). The role of community pharmacists in the care of drug misusers was seen as crucial, since they provided a significant point of contact as part of primary health care services, and generally had regular contact with patients. Hospital pharmacists too were seen to have an important role in advising general hospital clinicians when a patient maintained on substitute medication was admitted to hospital.

Government policy in relation to services for drug users continues to view pharmacy in a positive light. The role of community pharmacists in this area looks set to develop further as a result of the government's new national strategy for pharmacy (Anon, 2000). However, at the start of the twenty-first century the situation is changing rapidly, and policy in relation to the role of the community pharmacist remains fluid. It seems likely that the future will be determined as much by the actions and aspirations of pharmacists themselves as by the complex range of social, economic, political and technological factors which determine drug misuse, and society's response to it.

CONCLUSION

In this chapter, we have seen that changes in systems for the control of dangerous drugs did not transform patterns of supply and use overnight, or redefine professional boundaries in any dramatic way. Rather, they contributed to a slow process of change in attitudes to these substances, and a number of watersheds in this process can be identified. Initial systems for the control of substances liable to misuse were based on pharmaceutical regulation. But the 1920s were a significant watershed, with the Dangerous Drugs Act of 1920 heralding a shift to a medico-legal system of control.

A further time of boundary reconfiguration between "drugs" and "medicines" came in the 1960s with the Dangerous Drugs Act of 1965, and the subsequent Misuse of Drugs Act of 1971. Not only did the substances themselves become redefined but so also did those substances used in the treatment of substance abuse. The British National Formulary introduced a category of "drugs used in substance dependence" only in 1989, which included drugs used in alcoholism, cigarette smoking and opioid addiction, although the preparations involved had appeared elsewhere in the text for a number of years previously.

For the profession of pharmacy the story has been one of mixed fortunes, as the role of pharmaceutical regulation has waxed and waned. During the first half of the twentieth century it took a back seat to medical control, with its principal role as the dispensing of prescriptions. But in the last third of the twentieth century pharmacy has rebuilt its role. This has been dependent on three main changes: those that have occurred within the profession, those that have taken place in the nature of drug taking, and changes in conceptualisation and definition of drugs and medicines. These have been the three key themes of this chapter. But it has only been since the 1980s that community pharmacy has begun again to take a full role in tackling the complex issues that surround the misuse of drugs.

REFERENCES

Anderson SC, Berridge VS (2000a). The Role of the Community Pharmacist in Health and Welfare 1911 to 1986. In Bornat J, Perks RB, Thompson P, Wamsley J. (eds.) *Oral History, Health and Welfare, Routledge,* London, pp. 48–74.

Anderson SC, Berridge VS (2000b). Opium in Twentieth-Century Britain: Pharmacists, Regulation and the People, *Addiction*, 95, 2–6.

Anon (1981). What Future for General Practice Pharmacists? *Pharmaceutical Journal*, 227, 300–301.

Anon (2000). Plan Sets Out How Pharmacy Can Build a Future For Itself, Says Minister. *Pharmaceutical Journal*, 265, 397–400.

Berridge V (1980). The Making of the Rolleston Report 1908–1926. *Journal of Drug Issues*, 10, 7–28.

Berridge V (1996). *AIDS in the UK: The Making of Policy 1981–1994*, Oxford University Press, Oxford.

Berridge VS (1999). *Opium and the People,* Free Association Books, London.

Blenkinsopp A, Panton R (1991). *Drug Misuse, in Health Promotion for Pharmacists*, Oxford University Press, Oxford, 179–194.

Cherry P, Tredree R, Streeter H, Brain K (1986). The Development of an Addiction Treatment Service, *Pharmaceutical Journal*, 236, 329–31.

Data supplied by Pharmacy Practice Division (1998). Edinburgh.

Departments of Health (1999). *Drug Misuse and Dependence: Guidelines on Clinical Management*, The Stationery Office, London.

Downes D (1988). *Contrasts in Tolerance: Post War Penal Policy in the Netherlands and in England and Wales*, Clarendon Press, Oxford.

Gerrett D, Anderton D, Cullen AMS (1987). The Pharmacist's Role in Drug Abuse. *British Journal of Pharmaceutical Practice*, 9, 422–41.

Holloway SWF (1991). *Royal Pharmaceutical Society of Great Britain 1841 to 1991: A Political and Social History*, The Pharmaceutical Press, London.

Robertson R (1990). The Edinbugh Epidemic: A Case Study. In Strang J and Stimson G (eds.) *AIDS and Drug Misuse*, Routledge, London, pp. 95–107.

RPSGB (1988a). Guidelines for Pharmacists Involved in Schemes to Supply Clean Syringes and Needles to Addicts. *Pharmaceutical Journal*, 241, 253.

RPSGB (1988b). Sale of Hypodermic Syringes and Needles. In: *Medicines, Ethics and Practice: A Guide for Pharmacists*. Royal Pharmaceutical Society of Great Britain, London.

RPSGB (1992). *Pharmaceutical Care: The Future for Community Pharmacy*. The Royal Pharmaceutical Society of Great Britain, London.

RPSGB (1998). Report of the Working Party on Pharmaceutical Services for Drug Misusers. *Pharmaceutical Journal*, 260, 418–423.

RPSGB (2000). *Medicines, Ethics and Practice: A Guide for Pharmacists*. The Royal Pharmaceutical Society of Great Britain, London.

Scottish Home and Health Department (1975). *Misuse of Drugs in Scotland*, HMSO, Edinburgh.

Sheridan J, Strang J, Barber N, Glanz A (1996). Role of Community Pharmacies in relation to HIV Prevention and Drug Misuse: Findings from the 1995 National Survey in England and Wales. *British Medical Journal*, 313, 272–274.

Strang J, Sheridan J, Barber N (1996). Prescribing Injectable and Oral Methadone to Opiate Addicts: Results From the 1995 National Postal Survey of Community Pharmacies in England and Wales. *British Medical Journal*, 313, 270–272.

The Nuffield Foundation (1986). *Pharmacy: The Report of a Committee of Inquiry Appointed by the Nuffield Foundation*, The Nuffield Foundation, London.

Webster C (1996). *The Health Services Since the War Volume II: Government and Health Care, The British National Health Service 1958–1979*, The Stationery Office, London, p. 953.

Wingfield J, Evans V (1999). Reaching Agreement with Drug Misusers. *Pharmaceutical Journal*, 262, 131.

4

Reviewing the situation: pharmacists and drug misuse services in England and Wales

Janie Sheridan and John Strang

INTRODUCTION

There has been an increased awareness in recent years both by the Government and by the Royal Pharmaceutical Society (Department of Health, 1996; RPSGB, 1998) about the role that community pharmacists can play in providing services for drug misusers. The chapter will focus on a number of surveys conducted in England and Wales; readers will find detailed reviews of the evidence from Scotland and Northern Ireland in Chapters 5 and 6, respectively, whilst an international overview is given in Chapter 7.

In the six month period up to March 31st 2000 there were 31,800 contacts made with treatment services in England, an increase of 8% on the previous six months. The majority of these individuals reported opiates as their main drug of misuse (74%) (Department of Health, 2000), followed by stimulants and cannabis. Many of the individuals would be using community pharmacies as a source of clean injecting equipment or for collection of their prescribed treatments for substance misuse, e.g. methadone.

Historically, much of the detail of additional work and innovative practice of community pharmacists has gone uncharted and the contribution of pharmacists has often failed to be fully recognised by those within and outside the profession. However, pharmacy practice research carried out over the last decade has, to a great extent, revealed some of the picture to a wider audience. Practice research is not just about numbers and percentages, but also provides information on the implications for pharmacy practice, for drug misusers and for policy makers. In this chapter, the data from a national survey of England and Wales are firstly reviewed, and then data between the two countries are compared. Further sections then look at other research conducted at a more local level. The areas of practice which are reviewed include:

- dispensing of controlled drugs such as methadone
- supervised dispensing of methadone in the pharmacy
- sales of injecting equipment
- involvement in needle exchange schemes
- provision of advice.

The chapter also reviews the evidence relating to some of the problems faced by pharmacists.

There has been a continued rise in the numbers of drug users seeking treatment in England and Wales, as can be seen by the Home Office Addicts Index figures (see Figure 4.1). These data represent notifications by doctors for people who have sought treatment for drug-related problems with a number of drugs including heroin, methadone and cocaine. In 1988 there was a total of 12,644 notifications to the Home Office Addicts Index, compared to 43,372 in 1996 – the last year for which figures are available (Home Office, 1997). In 1988 – early in the history of harm reduction and HIV, a national postal survey of a random sample of one in four community pharmacies in England and Wales, stratified by health authority, was carried out through the National Addiction Centre in London. The survey found that almost one quarter of community pharmacists dispensed controlled drugs (CDs) to drug addicts, 28% sold needles and syringes to known or suspected drug injectors and 3% were involved in needle exchange (Glanz *et al.*, 1989). Since then, community pharmacy activities have been put under the microscope and we will now have a look at some of these results.

National survey of community pharmacies in England and Wales in 1995
In the mid 1990s the Department of Health commissioned a number of research projects to look at the effectiveness of services for drug users, to inform part of the Task Force Report (Department of Health, 1996). This included a re-examination study of pharmacies in England and Wales conducted using the same methodology as the 1988 study seven years earlier (Glanz *et al.*, 1989). It had been noted by pharmacists themselves that their involvement in service provision had increased, and this study provided the first real evidence for this (Sheridan *et al.*, 1996).

The survey addressed three key areas of service provision: dispensing CD prescriptions for the management of drug misuse, sales of sterile injecting equipment and involvement in needle exchange. The survey achieved a response rate of over 70% after four mailshots, giving a final sample size of 1984 pharmacies. With regard to dispensing CDs such as methadone, 50% of pharmacies were providing this service

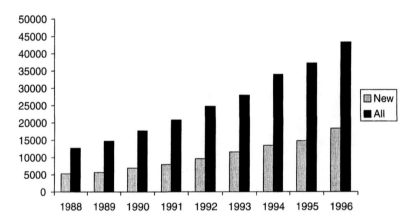

Figure 4.1 Addicts notified to the Home office. Home Office Statistics Bulletin issue 22/97 (1997).

to an estimated 40,000 clients. The mean number of clients per pharmacy was 5.9, with a range of 1–180 – most pharmacies only having one or two clients.

Pharmacists also provided information on the prescriptions they were dispensing for drug misuse at the time of completing the questionnaire. The vast majority were for methadone, of which approximately four fifths were for methadone mixture, 11% for tablets and 9% for ampoules. Other drugs being dispensed were amphetamine (mainly dexamphetamine), diamorphine and various other opioids and benzodiazepines.

Pharmacists were also asked to provide information about the distribution of clean injecting equipment, either through pharmacy sales or as part of free needle and syringe exchange schemes. With regard to sales from pharmacies, 31% of pharmacies had been asked to sell injecting equipment in the previous week, with a range of 1–180 requests per pharmacy estimated during this period. Thirty-five per cent of pharmacies were selling equipment, with a further 42% willing if there were local demand. With regard to participation in free needle exchange schemes, 19% of pharmacies provided this service, with a further 36% willing to do so if a scheme was set up in their area.

Figure 4.2 shows a comparison of the involvement in service provision in 1988 and 1995. The proportion of pharmacies providing a dispensing service had doubled during that time period, and while there had been only a small increase in the proportion currently selling injecting equipment, there had been a six-fold increase in the proportion involved in needle exchange schemes. This large increase can partly be explained by the fact that needle exchange in the UK was in its infancy in 1988 – the government pilot was conducted in 1987 (Stimson *et al.*, 1988) and support for this service and the willingness to become involved took some time to emerge.

Data from the Home Office Addicts Index around this time indicate that the number of drug addicts in contact with treatment had increased (Home Office, 1997), and Department of Health data on methadone prescription numbers indicated a significant increase in the prescribing of drugs in section 4.10 of the British National Formulary (Drugs used in Substance Misuse) (Department of Health, 1997). A comparison of the two studies revealed that not only had the proportion of pharmacies

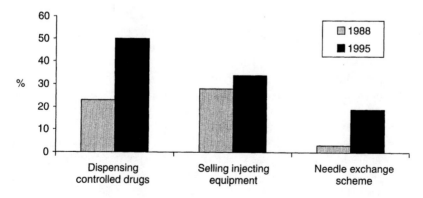

Figure 4.2 Community pharmacies in England and Wales: involvement in service provision for drug misusers in 1988 and 1995.

dispensing CDs such as methadone, doubled, but the mean number of clients at each service-providing pharmacy had also increased substantially; therefore more pharmacists were providing services to a greater number of clients. However, problems for community pharmacists often occur when they have too many methadone patients or needle exchange clients using the pharmacy, so the implications of a continued rise in client numbers needing pharmacy services are that unless more pharmacists are willing to provide some services, saturation point may be reached.

The survey also investigated pharmacists' attitudes towards service provision. Overall, respondents were in favour of a role for pharmacists in HIV prevention. However, they had concerns about the effect that drug users might have on their business and indicated a need for further training. In addition, a significant minority indicated that they would not easily be able to get support if they had a problem when working with drug users (Sheridan *et al.*, 1997). Further analysis of these data investigated the relationship between a pharmacist's attitudes towards service provision and whether or not they provided services. The study found an association between those with more positive (or less negative) attitudes and being involved in service provision.

A number of conclusions can be drawn from this study. The first is that community pharmacy has risen to the challenge of an ever increasing demand for methadone prescribing and supply of clean injecting equipment. However, if pharmacists are to continue to provide these services, they need to be provided with the support of prescribers and other members of the health care team, and to be trained in order that they feel competant and confident to provide services.

Welsh pharmacy and comparisons between England and Wales

Differences between England and Wales in the size of their drug misuse problems and in the geography of the two countries means that it is interesting to compare data from them (within the above study). While England had around 10,000 community pharmacies in 1995, Wales, occupying a much smaller area and with a proportionately even smaller population (48,900,000 in England versus 2,917,000 in Wales in 1995 – ONS, 1999) had only 700. Many of these pharmacies were in very rural locations. Drug problems in Wales at the time of the survey were different from those in England and Scotland, with evidence of a much larger amphetamine problem; in 1993 (the year for which most recent figures were available), seizures for amphetamines in Wales were 663 out of a total of 4,338 (15.3%) seizures of all drugs. This compares to 13.5% of all seizures in England and in Scotland for the same year (Home Office, 1994).

With regard to community pharmacy in Wales, a study in 1992 indicated that a number of pharmacies in all health authorities were providing clean injecting equipment through sales, were willing to take part in a needle exchange scheme and were willing to dispense methadone prescriptions.

Results from the 1995 national survey indicate that 80% of responding community pharmacists in Wales were very supportive of a role for community pharmacy in HIV prevention in the context of drug misuse, although 45% anticipated problems in the pharmacy when working with this client group, and 67% indicated a need for training. Two fifths (41%) of Welsh pharmacies were dispensing prescriptions for controlled drugs, fewer than in England, possibly reflecting a greater number of drug users in England and a larger opiate problem. Pharmacies dispensing CDs for drug misuse had a smaller mean number of clients per pharmacy (3.7) than those in England (6.0). Over one third (34%) were selling needles and syringes and 32% were involved in a needle exchange scheme, a far greater proportion than in England (18%); however similar proportions were unwilling to provide the service, indicating the possibility that more work had been done in encouraging Welsh pharmacists to become involved (Sheridan and Strang, 1998).

Providing needle exchange

Pharmacy-based needle exchange (PBNX) has developed at a local level, with little central guidance on the delivery of services and the manner in which they are monitored. This means that different schemes will have a variety of protocols and equipment provided will vary from scheme to scheme. Small-scale studies have looked at local service provision and user acceptance of needle exchange (Anthony *et al.*, 1995; Clarke *et al.*, 1998; Hollyoak and Wardlaw, 1992; Jayaratnan and Daff, 1993; Jones *et al.*, 1998; Rees *et al.*, 1997; Tucker, 1997).

On a larger scale, the scope and activities of pharmacists providing needle exchange has been studied in the south-east of England, from both the pharmacist and client perspective. At the time the study was conducted there were 440 participating pharmacies in PBNX in the former North and South Thames Regional Health Authorities in England. All pharmacies were sent a postal questionnaire to be completed by the pharmacist in charge of PBNX and after non-responder follow-up and telephone follow-up a response rate of 87% was obtained (Sheridan *et al.*, 2000).

The study investigated the types of equipment supplied by pharmacies across the schemes. All outlets provided 1 ml insulin syringes with a wide range of other equipment including other needles and barrels, personal sharps containers, swabs and leaflets. Many pharmacists reported being asked for other injecting paraphernalia (not supplied as part of the needle exchange scheme) such as citric or ascorbic acid, the supply of which is prohibited by law for use for the purposes of illicit drug taking (see Chapters 9 and 10).

Pharmacists were also asked about how they felt about providing needle exchange in the context of an organised scheme. The majority were satisfied with the way the service was run, would encourage others to join and were positive about one of PBNX's functions to put injectors in touch with help services. However, they did not believe injectors should be given advice unless they asked for it.

The study also investigated problems faced by pharmacists and their opinions on the level of support they were given. In general, pharmacists reported that the more serious problem of violence had *not* occurred in the previous 12 months, occurring only "rarely" or "never" in 83% of cases. Other problems such as shoplifting were more common, occurring "often" or "sometimes" in 45% of cases, and clients coming into the pharmacy intoxicated occurring "often" or "sometimes" in 30% of cases (see Figure 4.3). One quarter of pharmacists reported that they "always" or "sometimes" refused to carry out an exchange transaction when clients behaved disruptively.

Pharmacists were also asked to rate the adequacy of the support they were given in providing the service according to a number of domains, such as printed literature, supply and collection of injecting equipment, support from coordinator and support via training. Overall, most pharmacists were satisfied with the delivery and collection

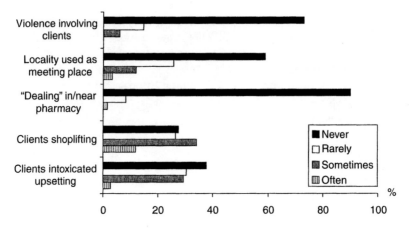

Figure 4.3 Incidents in the pharmacy needle exchange pharmacies.

Source: Sheridan J, Lovell S, Turnbull P, Parsons J, Stimson G, Strang J. (2000) Pharmacy-based needle exchange (PBNX) schemes in south east England: Survey of service providers. *Addiction*, 95, 1551–1560. www.tandf.co.uk. (with permission)

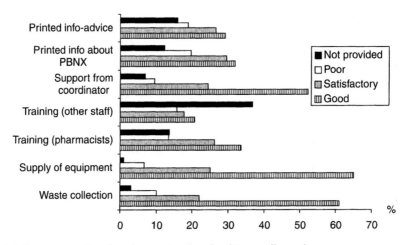

Figure 4.4 Support services for pharmacists involved in needle exchange.

of injecting equipment and also with the support of the coordinator of the scheme. However, they were less satisfied with other aspects such as printed materials about the service and with training (see Figure 4.4).

A number of local studies have been carried out into the provision of pharmacy needle exchange, some of which have described needle exchange schemes in the context of them being new and experimental initiatives. For example, Hollyoak and Wardlaw described a needle exchange scheme in the North East of England in 1992, and concluded that such a scheme was feasible, but that it needed to have the support of pharmacists, a clear but flexible policy, and an understanding of the needs of injecting clients. The authors also pointed out that while some problems had occurred with a small minority of clients, such as aggression and verbal abuse, overall there were few difficulties.

In 1993, McBride *et al.*, surveyed community pharmacists in Mid Glamorgan, Wales. They found a steady increase in the sales of injecting equipment, with injectors mainly buying 1 ml insulin syringes. Pharmacists were also found to be willing to take part in a tiered harm reduction service where, at the bottom tier pharmacists would provide information only, at the highest tier pharmacists would provide a full needle exchange service, thus allowing pharmacists to become involved at a level where they felt comfortable (McBride *et al.*, 1993).

Attitudes towards providing clean injecting equipment were studied by Rees *et al.* (1997), surveying community pharmacists in a health authority area of South East England. The research found that those willing to provide clean injecting equipment were significantly more likely to have positive attitudes towards supply, less likely to believe in negative outcomes of service provision (e.g. shoplifting) and that other pharmacy professionals would wish to make this service available. They recommended that those involved in service development should take note of incentives and disincentives to providing services in order to fully develop future services.

The views of clients of pharmacy needle exchanges were reviewed by Clarke *et al.*, (1998). The study looked at their opinions of the type and amount of equipment being given out as part of a needle exchange scheme in South East London. The study noted that while clients were generally satisfied with needle exchange pack contents, many would have preferred a service which allowed them to chose their equipment themselves, and there were a number of requests for additional equipment to be supplied, such as citric acid and water for injection-products which pharmacists were not allowed to provide due to legal restrictions.

Barriers to service provision
The national survey of community pharmacists (Sheridan *et al.*, 1996, 1997) investigated barriers to involvement in service provision. Pharmacists who were not providing services were asked to indicate their reasons for this. "No demand" was a frequent response; however, it is not possible to ascertain whether this was a true lack of demand i.e. no one was requesting the service, or whether as a result of an awareness that the pharmacist did not like providing the service, drug users had ceased to request it. In addition to a "lack of demand", a number of other themes emerged. Many of these were "client-related", such as client behaviour in the pharmacy (disruption, intoxication, threats of violence, and problems with clients attending accompanied by friends). Pharmacists also reported incidents of clients becoming agitated and disruptive when the pharmacist was unable to dispense a methadone prescription due to it being incorrectly written by the prescriber.

Lack of supplementary funding or financial recompense was also a barrier to service provision, with pharmacists reporting that the remuneration received for providing the services was not sufficient to cover their professional input or stock lost through shoplifting. In addition, a wide variety of service-related issues emerged as barriers such as the pharmacy being too small to stock needle exchange equipment, lack of staff, lack of time and the physical layout of the pharmacy being inappropriate. Some pharmacists also reported that they felt inadequately trained or lacked confidence when dealing with this client group. Negative attitudes, as previously stated, have been shown to be associated with non-involvement in service provision, and other studies of community pharmacists have noted similar attitudinal issues (Rees *et al.*, 1997; Harding *et al.*, 1992). Whether or not it is possible to effect a change in attitudes amongst those who stigmatise drug misusers and thus increase the pool of service providers remains a moot point.

There also exist, amongst service providers, certain barriers to an increased level of involvement in service provision. There is often an expectation among those specialising in drug misuse that generic health care professionals such as pharmacists should provide more in the way of services for their drug using clients, including the provision of advice and referrals to appropriate services. Research has shown that a significant proportion of pharmacists provide advice and have information leaflets on the premises (Sheridan *et al.*, 1996, 2000). However, research into needle exchange provision noted that pharmacists were unwilling to be proactive in providing information and advice, preferring to wait until asked by clients (Parsons *et al.*, 1999). For many pharmacists, the client seems to be the "expert" on drug misuse leaving them feeling disempowered with regard to the provision of guidance.

Supervised methadone
In many parts of the world, the supervision of the consumption of methadone in front of the pharmacist is the norm (see Chapter 12). However, little research has been carried out that looks at pharmacists' attitudes towards providing this service. In the national survey in England and Wales, 39% of community pharmacies indicated that they believed supervising the consumption of CDs in the pharmacy was an appropriate role for the community pharmacists (Sheridan *et al.*, 1997). Local pilot studies in London indicate that pharmacists experience few problems in providing this service and the majority of participating pharmacists were willing to continue to provide the service. Furthermore, in Glasgow, where supervised administration of methadone (SAM) is the usual way in which methadone is dispensed, 85% of the city's pharmacists provide this service. Studies have been carried out in Scotland looking at clients' views of SAM (Matheson *et al.*, 1999) and these are reported in Chapter 8. In the main, clients sometimes have issues around the attitudes of certain pharmacists towards them, and many report that lack of privacy is an issue.

How has research influenced practice and policy?
It is not possible to conclude definitively the extent to which practice research has influenced pharmacy practice and policy in England and Wales, although the Government has noted the contribution of the profession (Department of Health, 1996), recommending that pharmacists continue to provide needle exchange, and that other services such as supervised consumption should be further explored. Furthermore, the new Government clinical guidelines on the management of drug misuse fully recognise the role of pharmacy, the fact that it is an essential cog in the machinery of delivering treatment to drug users and the necessity for other professionals to collaborate closely with their community pharmacy colleagues (Departments of Health, 1999).

Research can have an impact on practice through informing service delivery, best practice, and describing barriers to service provision. Furthermore, research focussing on the views of clients provides essential data for service providers, purchasers and policy makers on the acceptability of services, their uptake and engagement of clients in continued service utilisation. Repeated surveys of community pharmacy activity, attitudes and barriers to service provision will enable purchasers and policy makers to recognise the impact of this branch of the profession on the management of drug misuse and to assess whether any "untapped potential" still exists.

REFERENCES

Anthony R, Shorrock PJ, Christie MM (1995). *Pharmacy based needle and syringe exchange schemes: an evaluation within Trent Region.* Nepenthe Press, Leicestershire Community Drug and Alcohol Teams.

Clarke K, Sheridan J, Williamson S, Griffiths P (1998). Consumer preferences amongst pharmacy needle exchange attenders. *Pharmaceutical Journal,* 261, 64–66.

Department of Health (1996). *The Task Force to review services for drug misusers – report of an independent review of drug treatment services in England.* The Stationery Office, London.

Department of Health (1997). *Statistics of prescriptions dispensed in the community: England 1986–1996.* London, Statistical Bulletin 1997/15.

Departments of Health (1999). *Drug Misuse and Dependence Guidelines on Clinical Management.* The Stationery office, London.

Department of Health (2000). *Statistics from the Regional Drug Misuse Databases for six months ending March 2000.* Department of Health, London.

Glanz A, Byrne C, Jackson P (1989). The role of community pharmacies in the prevention of AIDS among injecting drug misusers: findings of a survey in England and Wales. *British Medical Journal,* 299, 1076–1079.

Harding G, Smith FJ, Taylor KM (1992). Injecting drug misusers: pharmacists' attitudes. *Journal of Social and Administrative Pharmacy,* 9, 35–41.

Hollyoak VA, Wardlaw C (1992). A community pharmacy based needle exchange scheme. *Pharmaceutical Journal,* 249, 241–242.

Home Office (1994). *Statistics of drug seizures and offenders dealt with, United Kingdom, 1993.* Area Tables.

Home Office (1997). *Statistics of drug addicts notified to the Home Office, United Kingdom, 1996. Issue 22/97 14 October 1997.* Home Office, London.

Jayaratnan R, Daff C (1993). Newham Needle and Syringe Exchange Scheme. *Pharmaceutical Journal,* 251, 225–226.

Jones P, Van Teijlingen ER, Matheson CI, Gavin S (1998). Pharmacists' approach to harm minimisation initiatives associated with problem drug use: the Lothian survey. *Pharmaceutical Journal,* 260, 324–327.

Matheson C, Bond C, Hickey F (1999). Prescribing and dispensing for drug misusers in primary care: current practice in Scotland. *Family Practice,* 16, 375–379.

McBride AJ, Meredith-Smith RN, Davies NE (1993). Helping injecting drug users – a role for community pharmacists. *Pharmaceutical Journal,* 250, 708–709.

Office For National Statistics (1999). *Annual Abstracts of Statistics,* The Stationery Office, London.

Parsons J, Sheridan J, Turnbull P, Lovell S, Avendano M, Stimson G, Strang J (1999). *The implementation, development and delivery of pharmacy-based needle exchange schemes in north and south Thames,* The Centre for Research on Drugs and Health Behaviour, London.

Rees L, Harding G, Taylor KMG (1997). Supplying injecting equipment to drug misusers: a survey of community pharmacists' attitudes, beliefs and practices, *International Journal of Pharmacy Practice,* 5, 167–175.

RPSGB (1998). Working Party report: Services for drug misusers. *Pharmaceutical Journal*, 260, 418–423.

Sheridan J, Strang J, Barber N, Glanz A (1996). Role of Community Pharmacies in relation to HIV prevention and drug misuse: findings from the 1995 national survey in England and Wales. *British Medical Journal*, 313, 272–274.

Sheridan J, Strang J, Taylor C, Barber N (1997). HIV prevention and drug treatment services for drug misusers: a national study of community pharmacists' attitudes and their involvement in service specific training. *Addiction*, 92, 1737–1748.

Sheridan J, Strang J (1998). Community pharmacy in Wales: 1995 data on HIV prevention and drug misuse services. *Journal of Mental Health*, 7(2), 203–210.

Sheridan J, Lovell S, Turnbull P, Parsons J, Stimson G, Strang J (2000). Pharmacy-based needle exchange (PBNX) schemes in south-east England: Survey of service providers. *Addiction*, 95, 1551–1560.

Stimson GV, Alldritt L, Dolan K, Donoghoe M (1988). Syringe exchange schemes for drug users in England and Scotland. *British Medical Journal*, 296, 1717–1719.

Tucker RP (1997). Clients' awareness of AIDS-related risk factors and their perceptions of a pharmacy-based needle exchange scheme. *Journal of Substance Misuse*, 2(1), 31–35.

5

Drug misuse and community pharmacy in Scotland

Christine M Bond and Catriona Matheson

INTRODUCTION

Scotland has experienced a distinctive national and local drug problem, particularly over the latter quarter of the twentieth century. An understanding is required of the escalating nature of the problem and the services which have been established for the management of drug misuse, with particular emphasis on the contribution of community pharmacy to these services. The national Scottish survey, described in the second section, identifies and quantifies some key practice and attitudinal characteristics. Recent local developments in practice are then considered in the third section, building on some of the findings of the national survey, and other external events. In the final section the future role of services is considered.

In common with most other countries, drug misuse in Scotland is not a homogeneous problem. There are a wide range of drugs used, from cannabis to heroin and cocaine. Between 1975 and 1984 in Scotland, the number of those notified and receiving CDs for the treatment of their drug dependence rose from 58 to 137. These numbers are minimal compared to the numbers of 1027 in the Grampian[1] area alone in 1998/99. Between 1980 and 1986 Scottish notifications increased almost ninefold whilst they only doubled in the rest of the UK.

One of the features said to be distinctive about drug misuse in Scotland is the high level of injecting. The Ministerial Drugs Force reported that in the early 1990s there were 20,000 regular or occasional injectors in Scotland, equivalent to 392 per 100,000 of the population, compared to 173 per 100,000 for the rest of the UK (Scottish Office Home and Health Department, 1994). The figures for drug misuse have continued to rise such that in 1997 the SMR database (Scottish Drugs Misuse database) reported that 8573 new patients were registered in Scotland (Grampian Health Board, 1999). Of these, over half were using heroin as their main drug, over half (56%) were injecting and the majority of these were sharing injecting equipment (see Table 5.1).

---

[1] Grampian is a health board area in the north-east of Scotland. It has a population of approximately 550,000 of whom a third live in the city of Aberdeen. Much of the area is rural. There are pockets of deprivation but the overall socio-economic status of the population is above the Scottish average.

Table 5.1 Scottish Drugs Misuse Database figures for the 8573 new patients registered during the 12 months until 31st March 1998

Drug used	Number using	Number using as main drug
Heroin	5163	4360
Prescribed methadone	1539	1206
Other methadone	950	406
Other opiates	2123	831
Sedatives and tranquillisers	5138	770
Cannabis	2508	383
Other substances	3011	617
Injecting behaviour		
Percentage of individuals reporting injecting drug misuse	56%	
Percentage of individuals reporting sharing injecting equipment	54%	

The above-mentioned SMR database was set up in 1990 by the Scottish Office Home and Health Department; when an individual enters treatment, the health care professional interacting with the drug misuser completes a standard registration form for the drug misuser, with demographic information, medical details and drug taking behaviour.

The dangers from injecting are well known. As well as the spread of bloodborne diseases such as hepatitis B and C, the injecting drug misuser exposes him/herself to local site damage such as abscesses, ulcers and gangrene. The additional threat of HIV in the second half of the 1980s and through the early 1990s focused attention on the need to introduce harm reduction methods into the range of services provided and there was an increase in the provision of needle and syringe exchange schemes through either statutory or non-statutory services. Indeed the relatively slow rate of increase of HIV infections in Scotland (an average of 156 per year between 1990 and 1996) has been attributed, at least partly, to the health promotion initiatives, with the needle and syringe exchanges for drug misusers particularly highlighted (Scottish Office Department of Health, 1998). In contrast, whilst infections reported amongst intravenous drug misusers have declined, numbers amongst gay men and heterosexuals have been slowly increasing (Scottish Office Department of Health, 1998). The threat of other bloodborne diseases of greater infectivity such as hepatitis B and C, continues to be a major concern and numbers of new hepatitis B infections per week are currently increasing steadily in some areas of Scotland such as Grampian (Conaty, 1999).

Whilst drug misuse is a national issue, there are certain areas where prevalence is much higher than elsewhere. The worst areas are predictably around the major metropolitan areas such as Glasgow, Edinburgh, Aberdeen and Dundee. However there are also inexplicable pockets of drug misuse such as the north east fishing town of Fraserburgh. This relatively affluent community has attracted national media attention because of the high prevalence of illicit opiate and benzodiazepine drug use which was a similar level to its nearest city (Aberdeen) at approximately 2.0% of the population. This contrasts with the levels for other rural areas in Grampian of between 0.4 and 0.7% (Grampian Health Board, 1999).

The contribution of community pharmacy and the funding

As in the rest of the UK, there are two main areas in which community pharmacy can contribute: in the provision of clean injecting equipment and in the dispensing of drugs for the management of drug misuse, notably methadone. The remuneration structure for community pharmacy services in Scotland is different from England. Pharmacists are currently paid a professional fee of £18,900 per annum, plus a dispensing fee per item of 94.5p (Scottish Executive Health Department, 2001). In addition, under a relatively recent agreement certain services are remunerated separately under a system of devolved local budgets and contracts, which has facilitated different payments across Scotland, depending on locally determined need. These services include Drug Wastage, Services to Residential Homes, Needle and Syringe Exchange, and the dispensing of methadone. The methadone fee is only for the dispensing of a CD, and the instalment fee for daily dosing, and does not include a payment for supervising the self administration of methadone (see below).

As methadone became the established substitute drug treatment of choice for opiate dependency, there were increasing reports in Scotland of leakage of the prescribed methadone onto the "black market", as in other areas of the UK. It was believed that in order to optimise the benefits of the substitute practice the supervision of the taking of the methadone dose was essential and this was a role that community pharmacists could provide. In Greater Glasgow Health Board, the widespread involvement of community pharmacists in the supervised administration of methadone was seen as an example of good practice, with proven benefits (Gruer *et al.*, 1997; Roberts *et al.*, 1998), which other localities within Scotland have sought to emulate, finally remunerating the provision of the supervision service through an extension of the locally agreed contract.

Similarly, as the demand for needle and syringe exchanges grew, the previously nationally agreed single tier annual fee of £650 increasingly failed to reflect either workload *per se* or workload differentials across providers, and the fee for needle and syringe schemes was renegotiated. As well as providing a more realistic payment for community pharmacists, the locally agreed fees also enabled Health Board managers to set standards for the provision of the services, based on the fundamental requirements of the Code of Ethics (Royal Pharmaceutical Society of Great Britain, 2002) and the standards issued by the Scottish Department of the Royal Pharmaceutical Society.

One of the first areas in Scotland to react (with a network of exchange sites) to an early local rise in HIV/AIDS, purportedly due to needle sharing, was Lothian. Community pharmacists in this area responded to an appeal from the Health Board to provide a needle and syringe exchange service which resulted in a network of 26 pharmacy-based exchanges in addition to other needle exchange providers (Jones *et al.*, 1998).

SCOTTISH NATIONAL SURVEY 1996

The background

Community pharmacists may be the most frequently contacted, or indeed the only contact made between a drug misuser and a health care professional. However, whilst there was potential to build a treatment partnership between pharmacists and drug misusers which could promote the success of any intended care plan, results from a Scottish study of drug users (Matheson, 1998; Neale, 1999) indicated that pharmacists with a negative attitude may have a detrimental effect on the drug misuser. Clients' views on pharmacy services are covered in Chapter 8.

This first national survey of Scottish community pharmacies, carried out in 1996, sought data on whether pharmacists accepted current strategies, were prepared to become increasingly involved in service provision, what reservations, if any, they had and how these could be overcome. This study addressed a current gap in knowledge by providing baseline information on the level of involvement, motivation and attitudes which could be used to make comparisons across Health Boards, with possible explanatory associations; it also developed a validated instrument for future use to monitor trends.

The study objective was, therefore, to assess the current level of involvement of community pharmacists in providing services to drug misusers and to identify barriers to increased participation. The study was funded by a grant from the Chief Scientist Office, Scottish Home and Health Department (Bond *et al.*, 1995).

The method

The study used a combination of quantitative and qualitative methods. A questionnaire survey of all community pharmacy managers in Scotland provided quantitative data and telephone and face-to-face interviews, with a sub-sample providing in depth data on selected issues.

Preliminary content setting interviews were carried out with eight pharmacists in the Health Board areas of Grampian and Tayside. A semi-structured interview schedule was used which allowed pharmacists to discuss issues important to them regarding: drug misuse in general, the provision of services to drug misusers and the pharmacist's role. Pharmacists who were currently involved and those with little or no involvement were interviewed, based on local data.

The final questionnaire included enquiry about pharmacy demography, current involvement with drug misusers, training, attitudes, and willingness to take part in a follow up telephone interview. A combination of closed and open questions was used to gain factual information and attitudes were surveyed using a series of statements compiled from the content setting interviews. A five point Likert scale (strongly agree to strongly disagree) was used to grade the respondents' level of agreement with each statement. The questionnaire was piloted in a national random sample of 51 pharmacies, and after minor revisions mailed to the remaining 1091 community pharmacies across Scotland in October 1995. Because of the perceived sensitivity of some of the questions total anonymity of respondents was achieved by asking for an identifiable reply paid card to be posted back at the same time, but separately from, the unidentified questionnaire form. Thus non-responders could also be identified whilst maintaining anonymity. Up to three reminders were sent out to non-respondents. A covering letter explained that the questionnaire should be completed by the pharmacist who managed the pharmacy on a daily basis. Only one questionnaire was provided per pharmacy.

The questionnaire form asked for volunteers for follow up interviews. Sixty-five were selected from those volunteering, to reflect a range of experience, attitude, health board area, and type of pharmacy, thus minimising the potential for bias. Forty-five were interviewed by phone, the remainder being unavailable for a variety of reasons.

Summary of results

A summary of the key study results are presented in this chapter. For full results see Matheson *et al.*, (1999a,b), and Matheson and Bond (1999). The questionnaire response rate was excellent at 79% of pharmacies, and 26% volunteered for the follow up interviews.

Attitudes

A range of attitudes was evident from the levels of agreement expressed with the various statements, as shown in Table 5.2 (Matheson *et al.*, 1999b).

A combined score was created from the responses to the individual statements; a score above zero represented a positive (or less negative) attitude towards drug misusers and providing services for them, and a score below zero a negative (or less positive) attitude. The scores were tested for levels of association with various demographic characteristics of the community pharmacies. Respondents from the city areas had a significantly higher (more positive) attitude score (6.5) than either urban or rural pharmacies (3.4 and 3.1 respectively). There was no association between age, or type of business with attitude.

Service provision

The questionnaire sought information on service provision. On average only 9% of all respondents provided a needle and syringe exchange service, although as with most of the variables there was a wide range across Health Boards. Of the 784 respondents not providing a needle and syringe exchange service, some indicated that this was because of a lack of demand (n = 258; 32%); others did not consider the pharmacy to be an appropriate place (n = 28; 3.6%). A much larger number (55%) were prepared to sell needles or syringes.

The interview data indicated that pharmacists who provided an exchange service did so because of local need, a sense of professional responsibility, recognition that this was part of the pharmacists' "extended role", and an understanding of the need to prevent sharing of needles because of the risk of transmitting blood-borne disease. Deterrents to the provision of an exchange were reported to be concern for the safety of staff, the work load and the inadequate remuneration. Similarly factors contributing to the selling of needles and syringes were associated with the need for clean equipment to prevent the spread of blood-borne disease, and the professional opportunity to bring the drug misuser into contact with services. Factors deterring pharmacists from selling needles and syringes included the conflict between issuing clean needles but not taking back dirty returns, giving mixed messages to patients on a methadone programme, and being seen to promote drug misuse (Matheson and Bond, 1999).

Sixty-one per cent of the respondents were involved with dispensing of drugs for the management of drug misuse, and 55% of these dispensed methadone. Of the community pharmacies 19% were currently supervising methadone for at least some patients, and a further 14% were willing to do so if there were a demand (Matheson *et al.*, 1999a). There was great variation by Health Board. The rate of supervised consumption was highest in Glasgow at 70% of all prescriptions for methadone dispensed. In one area the rate was as low as 0.3%.

The daily management of patients receiving methadone also varied considerably. The laying down of ground rules to a new person was common practice (only

Table 5.2 Response to attitude statements by 864 responders

		strongly agree/agree (%)	uncertain (%)	strongly disagree/disagree (%)
1	I believe dispensing CD to drug misusers, as part of a maintenance programme, is part of a pharmacist's professional remit. (n = 862)	76.7	10.0	13.0
2	I believe supplying or selling needles/syringes to intravenous drug misusers will help reduce the spread of HIV. (n = 864).	68.8	18.2	13.1
3	I believe drug misusers visiting my pharmacy would endanger the safety of staff. (n = 863)	32.7	30.2	37.0
4	I believe it is appropriate for pharmacists to provide advice (written or verbal) to drug misusers on the management of drug misuse. (n = 860)	53.3	22.8	23.5
5	I have no sympathy for drug misusers. (n = 862)	23.8	19.9	56.0
6	I would never supervise the consumption of CD by drug misusers on my pharmacy premises. (n = 862)	26.7	16.9	56.2
7	I believe providing drug misusers maintenance doses of CD won't stop them using street drugs. (n = 862)	65.1	22.6	12.1
8	Drug misusers visiting my premises would have a damaging effect on business. (n = 860)	34.2	33.2	32.1
9	I believe needles and syringes should only be supplied to drug misusers through a syringe/needle exchange scheme. (n = 863)	73.1	8.8	18.1
10	I believe the community pharmacy is an appropriate place for a syringe/needle exchange scheme. (n = 864)	30.3	22.9	46.7
11	Widespread dispensing of CD to drug misusers affects the distribution of the global sum in community pharmacies. (n = 853)	37.2	51.6	9.9
12	I believe supervising the consumption of CD by drug misusers on the pharmacy premises is an appropriate role for the community pharmacist. (n = 864)	44.2	18.3	37.5
13	I believe CD should be dispensed to drug misusers through a central clinic rather than community pharmacies. (n = 856)	44.0	17.5	37.6
14	I believe supervising the consumption of CD by drug misusers prevents the illicit selling of these CD on the street. (n = 857)	58.8	12.6	27.8

#	Statement			
15	I would never provide advice (written or verbal) to drug misusers on the management of drug misuse. (n = 859)	11.3	20.6	67.5
16	I believe providing a syringe/needle exchange scheme is a good source of income for community pharmacies. (n = 858)	8.4	31.9	58.9
17	I believe drug misusers should only be prescribed CD if it is in reducing doses to help them "come off" drugs. (n = 857)	69.5	12.8	16.9
18	I believe that if drug misusers ask to buy needles or syringes it indicates they are taking some responsibility for their health. (n = 857)	54.0	24.7	20.6
19	I believe the community pharmacy is not an appropriate place for a syringe/needle exchange. (n = 857)	48.6	18.5	32.1
20	I believe it is unethical to sell drug misusers needles or syringes. (n = 859)	16.8	19.4	63.2
21	I believe dispensing CD to drug misusers is a good source of income for those pharmacies which dispense CD. (n = 856)	41.4	23.8	33.8
22	I believe providing drug misusers maintenance doses of CD will stop them using street drugs. (n = 857)	15.4	24.7	59.1
23	I believe providing maintenance doses of CD to drug misusers is a waste of NHS resources. (n = 857)	23.1	26.2	49.9
24	I would never provide advice (written or verbal) on safer injecting to intravenous drug misusers. (n = 859)	29.1	21.6	48.8
25	I believe CD should be dispensed to drug misusers through community pharmacies rather than a central clinic. (n = 852)	33.1	20.5	45.0
26	I believe it is ethical to sell drug misusers needles or syringes. (n = 855)	54.1	23.6	21.1
27	I believe it is appropriate for pharmacists to provide advice to drug misusers on safer injecting. (n = 856)	46.3	25.5	27.5

7% never did), but conversely only 7% actually used a formal written contract. Eighty-four per cent of pharmacists made the prescription up in advance as a time saving measure and these pharmacists had a more positive attitude score. Three quarters believed that they treated drug misusers in the same way as other customers. Antisocial behaviour (violence, threats, abuse, shoplifting) had been experienced at some time by many of the pharmacists and 42% had withdrawn services from an individual patient on these grounds. Few pharmacists provided either written or verbal health promotion information.

The interviews illuminated this quantitative data. The majority of those pharmacists interviewed understood the principles behind the methadone maintenance programmes although some were concerned about its long term viability. It was reluctantly accepted as a practical option, although funding was a contentious issue. Pharmacists could feel isolated and unsupported, and the prescribing practices of some general practitioners were seen to be poorly controlled (Matheson and Bond, 1999).

The pharmacists involved in the provision of either a needle and syringe exchange or methadone dispensing had significantly higher (more positive – less negative) attitude scores than those who were not involved (Matheson *et al.*, 1999b).

Training
Over a quarter of the pharmacists responding had received training on drug misuse or the prevention of blood-borne diseases, with marked differences again in different Health Board areas (range 49% to <25%). Local seminars (50.5%) and the Scottish Centre for Postgraduate Pharmacy Education (SCPPE) courses (48%) were the most frequently mentioned source of training on drug misuse. Three quarters of the respondents wished for further training, with distance learning packages and local workshops being the most favoured format, and communication and counselling skills, information on drugs of misuse and the management of misusers being the most frequently suggested topics. About a fifth had never had, and did not want, training.

Misuse of "Over the Counter" (OTC) drugs
The pharmacists also reported in the questionnaire survey on OTC drugs those which they suspected were being misused. Seventy per cent of pharmacists felt that there was a problem in their area. The most frequently mentioned drug was Nytol, an antihistamine-containing product cited by 50% of the respondents. Opiate-containing products also featured heavily, particularly Kaolin and Morphine Mixture, Codeine Linctus, Feminax, Solpadeine, Paramol, Gee's Linctus, Night Nurse and Syndol. Sympathomimetic-containing products, such as Actifed or Do-Do tablets, featured to a lesser extent. Pharmacists identified potential OTC misuse through excessive requests from an individual, their suspicious appearance, or sudden increases in stock turnover. They tried to control the misuse by a range of methods including: suggesting the purchaser visited the doctor if their symptoms did not improve; keeping a record of sales requiring the name and address of the purchaser; only involving the pharmacist in the sales; refusing sales; removing the stock from the shelves; no longer stocking the product and alerting other pharmacists in the area. Those suspected of misusing OTC drugs were not necessarily in the traditional image of a drug misuser, and included the elderly and middle-aged women.

Conclusions and relevance of the study

The results indicated that those with a less positive attitude towards service provision for drug misusers were less likely to be involved in such services. If involved, those with a lower attitude score were less likely to consider the needs of the drug misusers as evidenced by their failure to make prescriptions up in advance or their treatment of drug misusers in the same way as other customers.

Pharmacists have some awareness of the public health issues associated with the service, but at different levels. Some have not fully considered the appropriate disposal side of selling needles, and are unsure of the relationship between prescribed methadone use and continued injecting. Provision of health promotion advice is rare, and largely reactive (Matheson *et al.*, 1999a). A more proactive approach could enhance the level of professional service provided in community pharmacies; fear may be a barrier to this.

There was also concern about the methadone programme at national and local levels. Pharmacists with established links to other providers, particularly the prescriber, were more positive, but others could feel unsupported and undervalued. The quality of the prescribing was another cause for concern for some pharmacists.

Training was an identified need, although not necessarily for the right people. Those with a more negative attitude may be less likely to attend such events. Although those with a positive attitude are more likely to provide services (Matheson *et al.*, 1999b), we cannot say whether the positive attitudes are the cause or the result of this greater involvement.

DEVELOPMENT IN PRACTICE

The national survey looked at attitudes and practice in relation to drug misusers. Three particular aspects are further developed below illustrated by local examples.

Training

Firstly, the national survey identified negative attitudes amongst practitioners towards drug misusers. It also linked these negative attitudes to those practitioners with less involvement in service delivery (Matheson *et al.*, 1999b). As emphasised above, it was not possible to say whether the negative attitudes were the result of little experience with this target group of patients, whether the negative attitudes had influenced a decision not to offer services to drug misusers or whether those with negative opinions had been involved in unpleasant experiences with drug misusers.

The survey identified a perceived wish for more training on topics related to drug misuse. These included topics in the affective domain such as communication skills and in the cognitive domain such as factual information on the drugs of misuse and on the management of drug misusers. Results of a small pilot which attempted to change attitudes were inconclusive, although some participants claimed they would change their future practice as a result of the training session.

Training in drug misuse is also an area identified as part of the core SCPPE programme. As well as the local courses they have provided national courses which have used the survey and follow up interviews described above as a focus for national training days and a distance-learning pack (Matheson *et al.*, 1999c).

Prescribing and dispensing of methadone
Secondly, the survey identified wide variations in workload associated with dispensing methadone. The repeat of the survey in Grampian after one year showed an increase in percentage of doses supervised by community pharmacists from 19 to 29%. Although this was encouraging, given the general acceptance of the need for supervised daily consumption of methadone, it was disappointing that this was still less than a third of all prescriptions. As well as community pharmacists indicating a reluctance to become involved, and therefore a minority of pharmacies bearing a disproportionate workload, there was a parallel situation emerging amongst general practitioners. Concern was expressed about lack of specialist medical support and inconsistent treatment, so that a range of substitute drugs was being prescribed, often without evidence of benefit, in large quantities and without sufficient patient assessment before prescribing.

In order to resolve both intra- and inter-professional issues amongst general practitioners and community pharmacists, a small group of representatives of both professions was convened. These were professionals actively involved in delivering the service on a day to day basis rather than office bearers of local groupings such as the Area Pharmaceutical Committee or the General Practice sub-committee of the Area Medical Committee. The group openly discussed problems encountered in practice and agreed ways to address these as shown in Table 5.3.

These then resulted in the mutual drawing up of agreed guidelines for the shared management of drug misusers subsequently known as the Shared Care Scheme because the guidelines supported consistent and integrated treatment across the specialist/general practice and general practice/community pharmacy interfaces. The guidelines sought to address all the concerns raised through local agreement as to the best management strategies. In practice the final guidelines, shown in Figure 5.1, (reproduced with kind permission of Grampian Health Board) although drawn up *de novo* were not dissimilar from other examples of good practice, for example in Greater Glasgow. However there was a feeling of local ownership of the guidelines which facilitated their local acceptance.

The guidelines were launched in April 1998 and the scheme was supported by the appointment of a Specialist Pharmacist in Drug Misuse. Since that time, the percentage of prescribed doses of methadone which are supervised has risen to 80%.

Needle and syringe exchanges
The national survey had also identified variation in professional practices relating to needle and syringe provision. This included participation in formal needle and syringe exchange schemes and the selling of needles. From a public health perspective, access to clean needles is an important issue, whilst complying with regulations and reassuring the public. There is little more emotive than a small child finding used needles in public places. In the last two years in Aberdeen alone there have been 15 such reports in the local press (Aberdeen Journals, 2000).

Once again local issues, such as the variation in needle and syringe exchange practice, are best resolved by face-to-face discussions to air and jointly address problems. Table 5.4 shows some of the problems highlighted in this way in Grampian and the means identified to address these. The group, originally formed to resolve local issues, continues to meet quarterly, supported by the local voluntary drugs agency,

Table 5.3 Examples of problems experienced by Grampian community pharmacists and general practitioners when providing substitute methadone

Problem	Resolution
SSAM not always enforced. Observed black market in street methadone. Inconsistent practice across GPs.	Guidelines for prescribing and dispensing to be developed and endorsed by local professional community pharmacy and general practice advisory committees, and adopted by practitioners.
GPs cannot find a pharmacist to provide SSAM. Pharmacists do not want new client expecting SSAM without opportunity to consider.	List of community pharmacists offering SSAM circulated to all GPs. GPs and patient to jointly identify a pharmacy of their choice, then contact them to ensure that the pharmacist will take this client on. Pharmacists have the option to decline.
No remuneration for SSAM.	Identification of new resource.
Community pharmacists aware of clients defaulting, using on top, selling on.	Formal acknowledgement of the community pharmacy as a member of the care term. Empowerment to contact GP with information about the client if professional judgement deems this appropriate. Drug misuser made aware of this at the start of the programme.
Pharmacists not always sure of the identity of the drug misuser. Fear of giving dose to an impostor.	Photos of drug misusers on regular scripts retained in pharmacy. Polaroid cameras made available to general practitioners and community pharmacists to facilitate this.
Drug misusers not aware of code of behaviour. Problems with shoplifting groups of drug misusers, threatening behaviour.	Contracts to be signed with pharmacy.
Community pharmacists cannot contact prescriber in the event of a prescription query.	Guaranteed access to prescriber through receptionist or hotline phone number.
Lack of knowledge.	Joint training with GPs and community pharmacists.
Lack of a forum to air problems.	Joint meeting with GPs and community pharmacists.

SSAM – Supervised self-administration of methadone.

GHB - Shared Care Scheme

Action Plan for GPs and Community Pharmacists when prescribing "substitute" medication for drug misusers

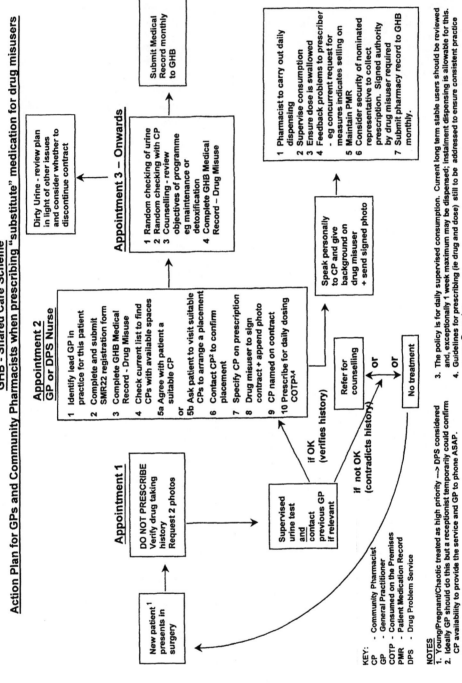

Appointment 1

DO NOT PRESCRIBE
Verify history
Request 2 photos

New patient [1] presents in surgery

Supervised urine test and contact previous GP if relevant

if OK (verifies history)

if not OK (contradicts history)

Refer for counselling

or

No treatment

Appointment 2
GP or DPS Nurse

1 Identify lead GP in practice for this patient
2 Complete and submit SMR22 registration form
3 Complete GHB Medical Record - Drug Misuse
4 Check current list to find CPs with available spaces
5a Agree with patient a suitable CP
   or
5b Ask patient to visit suitable CPs to arrange a placement
6 Contact CP[2] to confirm placement
7 Specify CP on prescription
8 Drug misuser to sign contract + append photo
9 CP named on contract
10 Prescribe for daily dosing COTP[3,4]

Speak personally to CP and give background on drug misuser + send signed photo

Appointment 3 – Onwards

1 Random checking of urine
2 Random checking with CP
3 Counselling - review objectives of programme eg maintenance or detoxification
4 Complete GHB Medical Record – Drug Misuse

Dirty Urine - review plan in light of other issues and consider whether to discontinue contract

Submit Medical Record monthly to GHB

1 Pharmacist to carry out daily dispensing
2 Supervise consumption
3 Ensure dose is swallowed
4 Feedback problems to prescriber - eg concurrent request for measures indicates selling on
5 Maintain PMR
6 Consider security of nominated representative to collect prescription. Signed authority by drug misuser required
7 Submit pharmacy record to GHB monthly.

KEY:
CP - Community Pharmacist
GP - General Practitioner
COTP - Consumed on the Premises
PMR - Patient Medication Record
DPS - Drug Problem Service

NOTES
1. Young/Pregnant/Chaotic treated as high priority —> DPS considered
2. Ideally GP should do this but a receptionist temporarily could confirm CP availability to provide the service and GP to phone ASAP.
3. The policy is for daily supervised consumption. Current long term stable users should be reviewed and, exceptionally 1 week maximum may be dispensed; instalment dispensing is allowable for this.
4. Guidelines for prescribing (ie drug and dose) still to be addressed to ensure consistent practice across Grampian.

Figure 5.1 Grampian Shared Care guidelines for managing drug misuse.

Table 5.4 Examples of some of the problems experienced by needle and syringe providers and ways identified to resolve these

Problem	Resolution
Lack of consistency of number of needles issued across providers. Aggressive pressure from drug misusers to issue more than allowed amounts "because everyone else does".	Posters detailing regulations for needle exchanges displayed by all providers.
Feeling of isolation in community pharmacy. Lack of confidence in handling difficult situations.	Formation of local support group with regular meetings. Support from Drugs Action staff. Training in handling difficult situations.
Lack of knowledge about other local resources.	Leaflets and posters for display and distribution.
Lack of knowledge about drug misuse.	Training from local drug workers.
Lack of knowledge about blood-borne diseases.	Training from Infectious Disease nurse.
Fear of contracting a blood-borne disease from accidental needle stick injury.	Hepatitis B immunisation for all staff in any needle exchange. Provision of chain mail gloves to handle used works. Guidance on spillages.
Service under-resourced.	Identification of additional money to remunerate the busier exchanges.
Lack of privacy for exchange, upset of other customers.	Support for creation of separate consultation area.
Fear of the drug misuser.	Panic buttons installed linked to the police. CCTV installed.

Drugs Action, and the Health Board. As is often identified, pharmacists are relatively isolated professionals and they benefit greatly from the discussion of issues, particularly in sensitive or contentious areas such as interactions with drug misusers where security, confidentiality and personal violence may all be involved.

Although personal safety, and security of retail stock, is often seen as an issue when considering participation in the provision of these services, and anecdotally reported as deterring participation, in practice these events are relatively rare as was demonstrated in a small local prospective survey (Lochrie *et al.*, 1997).

One further issue is the need to continually review evidence and ensure that the most clinically effective and cost effective treatments are being used. The principles of the shared care methadone guidelines developed in Grampian were corroborated by the recently revised *Clinical Guidelines for the treatment of Drug Misuse*, known as the 'Orange Guidelines' issued by the Scottish Office and Department of Health in England (Scottish Office, 1999). In particular these reiterated that methadone is the only treatment for which there is a substantial body of research evidence of benefit, that it should when appropriate be prescribed by general practitioners with specialist support (as opposed to specialists only), that community pharmacists have a key role, and that for at least the first three months of its administration it should be supervised. It further reminded clinicians of the fact that other drugs sometimes used as substitute drugs in drug dependency treatments, such as dihydrocodeine, are not licensed for this indication and should not be a first line option.

FUTURE IMPLICATIONS

The drug misuse situation is a dynamic one which needs continual monitoring and review. We have given in this chapter several examples of local problems which have been resolved by open debate, consensus and team-working across and within professions. In particular we have illustrated the potential contribution that community pharmacy can make, and welcome the support of this role by the Royal Pharmaceutical Society of Great Britain. The role of community pharmacy also needs to be supported locally by Health Boards through adequate remuneration and further support for premises modifications such as increased security, CD storage arrangements and private consulting areas.

However as demand increases, local solutions will continually be required to provide additional ways of providing traditional community pharmacy services, and alternative models of care may need to be developed. These might involve pharmacy outposts in non-community pharmacy outlets (e.g. health centres, community hospitals), dedicated drugs workers based in community pharmacies, or even innovative options such as a methadone bus which is already operating in one area in England. Even more unthinkable options such as methadone dispensing machines may need to be considered to meet the demand.

Finally the drug misusers' needs should always be considered in the development of new services. Although these may be difficult to obtain this should not mean that they are ignored, any more than any other patients group's views should be ignored. As shown in Chapter 8 this population of community pharmacy users have strong and important views as to the service they require and the effect of that service on the outcomes of their care. For this reason if for no other, participation in schemes for drug misusers is something which we cannot enforce on all pharmacists. Those with negative attitudes will rarely provide effective care; the mission should be to change attitudes, and thus increase participation.

REFERENCES

Aberdeen Journals (2000). Archives of *Press and Journal* and *Evening Express*, 1998–1999, Aberdeen.

Bond CM, Matheson C, Hickey F (1995). *Community pharmacists involvement with drug misusers: a Scottish national survey of pharmacists attitudes and practice/ Health Services and Public Health Research Committee.* Chief Scientist Office, The Scottish Home and Health Department K/OPR/2//2/D258.

Conaty S (1999). Consultant in Infectious Diseases, Grampian Health Board. Personal Communication.

Grampian Health Board (1999). *Annual Public Health Report.* Grampian Health Board, Aberdeen.

Gruer L, Wilson P, Scott R, Elliott L, Macleod J, Harden K, Forresterm E, Hinshelwood S, McNulty H, Silk P (1997). General practitioner centred scheme for treatment of opiate dependent drug injectors in Glasgow. *British Medical Journal*, 314, 1730–1735.

Jones P, van Teijlingen E, Matheson C, Gavis S (1998). Pharmacists' approach to harm minimisation initiatives associated with problem drug use: the Lothian survey. *Pharmaceutical Journal*, 260, 324–327.

Lochrie E, Bond C, Matheson C (1997). *The needle and syringe exchange service in Grampian: a review*. Department of General Practice and Primary Care, University of Aberdeen, Aberdeen.

Matheson C (1998). Views of illicit drug users on their treatment and behaviour in Scottish Community pharmacies: implications for the harm reduction strategy. *Health Education Journal*, 57, 31–41.

Matheson C, Bond CM (1999). Motivations for and barriers to community pharmacy services for drug misusers. *International Journal of Pharmacy Practice*, 7, 256–263.

Matheson C, Bond CM, Hickey FM (1999a). Prescribing and dispensing for drug misusers: current practice in Scotland. *Family Practice*, 16, 375–379.

Matheson C, Bond CM, Mollison J (1999b). Attitudinal factors associated with community pharmacists' involvement in services for drug misusers. *Addiction*, 94, 1349–1359.

Matheson C, Neale J, Roberts K, McCreadie M, Gourlay Y (1999c). *Pharmaceutical Care of the Drug Misuser: part A*, Scottish Centre for Post qualification Pharmaceutical Education, Strathclyde University, Glasgow.

Neale J (1999). Drug users' views of substitute prescribing conditions. *International Journal of Drug Policy*, 10, 247–258.

Roberts K, McNulty H, Gruer L, Scott R, Bryson S (1998). The role of the Glasgow pharmacist in the management of drug misuse. *International Journal of Drug Policy*, 9, 187–194.

Royal Pharmaceutical Society of Great Britain Working Party (2002). *Medicines, Ethics and Practice: A guide for pharmacists*, Royal Pharmaceutical Society of Great Britain, Issue 26, pp. 90–91, 99–100.

Scottish Executive Health Department (2001). *Scottish Drug Tariff*, Scottish Executive Health Department, Edinburgh.

Scottish Office Department of Health (1998). *Working together for a Healthier Scotland, A consultation document*. HMSO: CM3584.

Scottish Office (1999). *Clinical Guidelines for the treatment of Drug Misuse*. HMSO, Edinburgh.

Scottish Office Home and Health Department (1994). *Drugs in Scotland: meeting the challenge. Report of the Ministerial Drugs Force*, The Scottish Home and Health Department, Edinburgh.

6

Drug misuse in Northern Ireland: the role of the community pharmacist

*Glenda F Fleming, James C McElnay
and Carmel M Hughes*

BACKGROUND

Traditionally, Northern Ireland is recognised as having a lower incidence of illicit drug use when compared with other parts of the UK; however, the problem is now regarded as increasing (Department of Health and Social Services, 1995; Northern Ireland Drugs Campaign, 1999). As with other areas of the UK, it is difficult to obtain an accurate picture of the incidence, prevalence and type of drug abuse in Northern Ireland. A variety of sources, for example, official police (Royal Ulster Constabulary – RUC) and Department of Health statistics and surveys of the general population, are used to assess changes which have occurred. Summaries of the available information for Northern Ireland are presented in *Drug Strategy for Northern Ireland* (Northern Ireland Drugs Campaign, 1999) and *Illicit Drug Use in Northern Ireland: a handbook for professionals* (Health Promotion Agency for Northern Ireland, 1996).

The most commonly abused drugs in Northern Ireland are cannabis and ecstasy, with the use of heroin and cocaine considered low (Health Promotion Agency for Northern Ireland, 1996). The low use of heroin and cocaine is reflected in the number of registered addicts in Northern Ireland (Figure 6.1). The numbers are much lower than in other parts of the UK; for example in 1994, after adjusting for population, the number of notified addicts in Great Britain exceeded that in Northern Ireland by a ratio of 11:1 (Department of Health and Social Services, 1995). However, there is concern regarding the scale of the increase in the number of notified addicts observed in recent years.

The increasing trend of drug use is also reflected in drug seizures by the police (Table 6.1). It should be noted that while seizures of cannabis and ecstasy are high, seizures of heroin have remained relatively low. In recent years, resources available to the RUC for drug enforcement have increased, as explained by the Chief Constable in his 1995 report "... *in recognition of the growing drug problem in Northern Ireland, the number of officers in the (Drugs) Squad has been increased and new Squad offices have been opened*...". This increased resource was made possible by the cease-fires announced by the major terrorist organisations in Northern Ireland in 1994. It has been suggested that increases in drug seizures reflect changes in policing

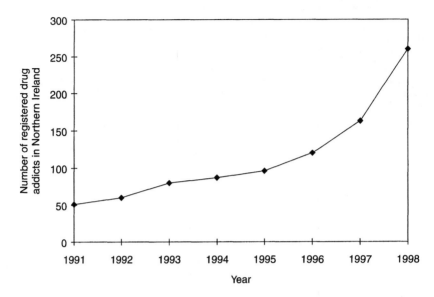

Figure 6.1 The number of notified addicts in Northern Ireland between 1991 and 1998.

Adapted from: Department of Health and Social Services, 1995; Health Promotion Agency for Northern Ireland, 1996; Northern Ireland Drugs Campaign, 1999.

rather than an increase in illicit drug misuse (McEvoy *et al.*, 1998). However, most commentators feel that there is also an increasing trend toward drug use in the region.

Further evidence for an increasing drug problem can be found in surveys of the general public, which include the Health Behaviour of School Children Surveys conducted by the Health Promotion Agency in conjunction with the World Health Organisation in 1992, 1994 and 1998. These surveys revealed that the number of fifth form pupils (average age 15 years) who had been offered illegal drugs increased from 25.5% in 1992 to 52% in 1998 (Northern Ireland Drug Campaign, 1999). The proportion of fifth form pupils reporting that they were using drugs at the time of the survey increased from less than 6% in 1992 to 18% in 1994 (Health Promotion Agency for Northern Ireland, 1995). A separate survey conducted by Craig (1997), funded by the Department of Education and the Health Promotion Agency for Northern Ireland, considered the views of older teenagers. The proportion of this sample (average age 16.5 years) that had been offered drugs was 63%. Only 2% of this sample thought that obtaining drugs would be difficult.

CHANGING DRUG POLICY IN NORTHERN IRELAND

The drug policies in Northern Ireland take account of national government strategies; however they are adapted to reflect the local situation. As the problem of drug abuse has evolved in the region, changes in policy have been observed.

In 1986, the illicit drug misuse problem in Northern Ireland was considered to be negligible and public education and prevention strategies were kept low-key, so as not to encourage experimentation (Department of Health and Social Services, 1995). Inevitably as the problem increased, the policy had to change, thus in 1995,

Table 6.1 RUC drug seizures 1992–1999

	1992[1]	1993[1]	1994[1]	1995[1]	1996/97[2]	1997/98[2]	1998/99[2]
Cannabis							
Kilograms	15.75	44.5	97	161.1	220.0	452.1	434.3
Plants	0	0	66	634	91	167	110
Joints (reefers)	0	0	0	0	338	186	163
Oil (gm)	0	0	0	0	0	1	0
Ecstasy							
Grams	0	0	0	0	103	26	112
Tablets	4408	2923	23,953	136,860	94,792	85,600	163,023
Capsules	0	0	0	0	50	169	122
Opiates							
Grams (all opiates)	20	363	34	8	190	144	231
Grams (heroin only)	Not available	Not available	Not available	Not available	189.5	143.3	227.5
Heroin liquid formulations (mls)	0	0	0	0	0	0	126
Heroin wraps	0	0	0	0	1	0	6
Morphine tablets	0	0	0	0	1242	1104	968
Morphine ampoules	0	0	0	0	5	0	0
Pethidine tablets	0	0	0	0	21	0	110
Pethidine ampoules	0	0	0	0	30	20	0

Adapted From:
1 Northern Ireland Drugs Campaign, 1998.
2 Royal Ulster Constabulary (RUC) Central Statistics Unit, personal communication.

"Drug Misuse in Northern Ireland: A Policy Statement" (Department of Health and Social Services, 1995) was published. In its statement of purpose, this document stated that:

The aim of policies and programmes in Northern Ireland to tackle drug misuse should be to reduce the acceptability and availability of drugs to young people and to reduce the health risks and other harm resulting from drug misuse by:

- Delivering an effective education and prevention programme
- Providing effective care, treatment and rehabilitation services for those using illicit drugs
- Vigorously pursing law enforcement, and ensuring the safety of communities from drugs and drug related crime.

In order to achieve these aims, five priorities were highlighted:

i. Education and prevention
ii. Treatment and rehabilitation
iii. Law enforcement
iv. Information and research
v. Monitoring and evaluation.

At around the same time, the Central Co-ordinating Group for the Action Against Drugs (CCGAAD), under the chairmanship of the Minister of State for Northern Ireland, was established (Department of Health and Social Services, 1995). This group promotes a co-ordinated approach in the fight against drugs and in 1996 launched the Northern Ireland Drugs Campaign, the main features of which are information, education, research and the development of drug co-ordination teams based in the health boards (Northern Ireland Drugs Campaign, 1999).

In 1998, a review of the existing policy in Northern Ireland led to the publication of an updated statement: *Drug Strategy for Northern Ireland* (Northern Ireland Drugs Campaign, 1999). It established four aims:

i. To protect young people from the harm resulting from illicit drug use
ii. To protect communities from drug-related anti-social and criminal behaviour
iii. To enable people with drug problems to overcome them and live healthy, crime-free lives
iv. To reduce the availability of drugs in communities.

This strategy is due for review in 2002.

DRUG MISUSE IN NORTHERN IRELAND: FACTORS AFFECTING THE SCALE OF THE PROBLEM

There are many theories regarding the reasons for a lower level of drug misuse in Northern Ireland (Murray, 1994). One major factor that has been identified revolves around the complex political situation in the region (McEvoy *et al.*, 1998). Terrorist groups on both sides of the political divide have been involved in a policing role against "anti-social behaviour" (including drug dealing) within their respective communities and indeed at one stage, several suspected drug dealers were murdered by an organisation calling itself "Direct Action Against Drugs".

In addition, the political situation led to a higher security force and police presence than in other regions of the UK. Murray (1994) suggests that this high level of visible policing and security force surveillance acted as a deterrent to the supply and distribution of illicit drugs. Murray (1994) also suggests that Northern Ireland in general is a conservative, law-abiding country. Non-terrorist crime is low and organised crime groups involved in drug running have not had a presence in the region. He also comments that the Church has a greater influence in Northern Ireland than in other parts of the UK and that close family and neighbourhood networks often exist; these factors have also mitigated against proliferation of illicit drug abuse.

With developments in the political environment, changes in many of the factors described above are occurring. This in turn will influence the evolving drug scene in the region.

SERVICE PROVISION AND POLICIES FOR DRUG MISUSERS

Because of the unique problems in Northern Ireland, service provision for drug misusers had been somewhat limited in comparison to the rest of the UK. The major differences are as follows:

Needle exchange

A needle exchange pilot started in eight pharmacies in Northern Ireland in March 2001. This scheme is still operating at the eight sites, although it is now out of the pilot phase.

Methadone prescribing

At this time, the Northern Ireland Protocol for Opiate Detoxification (Clinical Resource Efficiency Support Team, 1999) actively discourages methadone prescribing. General Practitioners (GPs) are advised to contact specialist services if they feel that methadone treatment is required. Normally methadone will only be offered by the specialist service in an in-patient setting, in cases of acute withdrawal. Partly as a result, community pharmacists and other members of the primary healthcare team have little contact with such patients.

Notification of addicts

In Northern Ireland, The Misuse of Drugs (Notification and Supply to Addicts) (Northern Ireland) Regulations, 1973, require doctors to notify the Chief Medical Officer of the Department of Health and Social Services if they suspect a patient is addicted to any of the fourteen notifiable CDs. In England and Wales, this requirement has been abolished in favour of voluntary reporting to regional drug misuse databases, but in Northern Ireland it has been retained.

Treatment services

Treatment services in Northern Ireland are centralised to specialist centres, with a lack of community involvement. There are a number of support organisations, mainly in the voluntary sector, but they primarily offer advice and counselling rather than active treatment. Most health-care professionals have little active involvement in this area, but due to changes in drug misuse trends, this may need to alter in the future. One member of the primary health-care team, who is in a position to contribute to management and control of drug misuse is the community pharmacist.

THE COMMUNITY PHARMACISTS' INVOLVEMENT IN HARM-REDUCTION PROGRAMMES

The National Addiction Centre in London has conducted research into the community pharmacists' role in drug misuse and HIV prevention, in England and Wales, in 1995 (Sheridan *et al.*, 1996) and found evidence of a major increase in use of community pharmacy services by drug misusers (see Chapter 4). Given the lower incidence of injecting drug use in Northern Ireland, it was anticipated that community pharmacists would have little contact with such users. In order to test this hypothesis, research similar to that in England and Wales has recently been undertaken in Northern Ireland.

In performing this research, minor amendments were made to the above mentioned questionnaire in order to make it applicable to the Northern Ireland setting. The questionnaire consisted of seven sections and included sections relating to: prescription details of (CDs) for clients who were receiving them for addiction/misuse; provision of needles to drug misusers (sales and needle exchange); opinion on services provided to drug misusers and the role of the pharmacist in drug misuse and HIV prevention.

The questionnaire was mailed on two occasions, to all community pharmacies in Northern Ireland (n = 507) and a final reminder letter was sent to pharmacies with their medical deliveries. A response rate of 67.5% (n = 342) was achieved in Northern Ireland, comparable to the response rate achieved in England and Wales (see Chapter 4). The results in Northern Ireland were strikingly different from those found in England and Wales (Chapter 4) or in Scotland (Chapter 5).

In Northern Ireland, only 9.7% (n = 33) of pharmacists reported dispensing CDs for the treatment of addiction/misuse; only nine patients were reported (by the 100% sample) to be receiving methadone. The most common reason for not dispensing CDs for addiction/misuse was lack of demand. In comparison, 50.1% of respondents in England/Wales (n = 992) were dispensing CDs for the treatment of addicts, with 3693 methadone prescriptions being identified by the one in four sample (Strang *et al.*, 1996).

The majority of respondents in Northern Ireland (71.6%) had never been asked to sell needles to known/suspected drug misusers. Of those who had, 17.7% had been asked to sell needles in the previous week; in England/Wales, 31% had received such requests. The majority of respondents in Northern Ireland (60.2%) reported that they would be prepared to sell needles if there was a demand.

As stated earlier, no needle-exchange scheme currently exists in Northern Ireland. However, 77.2% of the respondents indicated that they would be willing to participate if such schemes were introduced. In England and Wales, 18.9% of the respondents reported participation in needle-exchange schemes.

Pharmacists in Northern Ireland who were not willing to sell needles or participate in needle-exchange were asked to give reasons. These included ethical objections, business concerns (e.g. fear that addicts may damage regular trade) and safety reasons (e.g. concern regarding increased threat of attack).

Pharmacists in Northern Ireland were also asked a series of questions to assess their personal opinion on a variety of other services for drug misusers. Overall, few were currently providing services, but most would be willing to do so. The statements provided and the responses given are presented in Table 6.2.

To evaluate opinions on the role of the community pharmacist in relation to drug misuse and HIV prevention, pharmacists were asked to comment on a series of statements (Table 6.3). Overall, respondents agreed that they had an important role to play concerning drug misuse and the prevention of HIV. Opinion was, however, divided on a number of issues, for example, with regards to the pharmacist's role in the supervision of consumption of CDs. It was also evident that a large number of pharmacists were undecided on some issues; for example 44% neither agreed nor disagreed with the statement relating to drug misusers visiting the premises and the possible impact that this might have on their business. This section of the survey highlighted a need for training with over 90% of respondents indicating they needed training on how to deal with drug misusers who may visit their premises. Further questioning revealed that only 18.1% had received training on drug misuse and only 8.0% reported having received training on HIV prevention. In many cases, the training received was limited to undergraduate teaching at university. In addition, the majority of respondents were unsure or disagreed with the statement that if they needed to they could find someone to help with problems they may experience when dealing with drug misusers.

THE PHARMACISTS' ROLE – PRESENT AND FUTURE

Overall, the survey indicated that, at present, community pharmacists in Northern Ireland have little contact with injecting drug users. This is as expected, given the

Table 6.2 Activities and views of community pharmacists in relation to Northern Ireland on service provision to drug misusers

	Number of respondents to statement	Percentage of respondents		
		Currently do	Would be willing	Would not be willing
Have a sharps box on the premises	334	24.2	55.7	20.1
Accept equipment already in misusers' sharps box	331	1.8	70.4	27.8
Supply users with a personal sharps container	334	0.3	83.5	16.2
Supply information leaflets concerning drug misuse and HIV	334	23.4	74.8	1.8
Offer face-to-face advice concerning drug misuse and HIV prevention	330	3.0	83.1	13.9
Offer advice on treatment of drug misuse	331	4.2	84.0	11.8
Refer misusers to specialist agencies	336	2.1	94.0	3.9

Table 6.3 Opinions of Northern Ireland community pharmacists on the role of the community pharmacist in relation to drug misuse and HIV prevention

	Number of respondents to statement	Percentage of respondents				
		Strongly agree	Agree	Neither agree nor disagree	Disagree	Strongly disagree
The community pharmacist has an important role to play concerning drug misuse and the prevention of the spread of HIV	338	26.9	53.0	14.2	4.7	1.2
I need training in how to deal with drug misusers who may visit my premises	339	42.5	49.0	6.8	1.2	0.5
Drug misusers visiting my premises are likely to have a damaging effect on my business	339	13.3	28.9	44.0	12.6	1.2
I would be prepared to give injecting equipment to drug misusers if this was provided to me free of charge	337	10.4	53.4	17.8	12.5	5.9
I do not think that supplying injecting equipment to injecting drug misusers is an appropriate role for the community pharmacist	338	7.1	12.1	25.1	45.9	9.8
If I needed to, I could easily find someone to help me with any problems I might have when working with drug misusers	338	2.7	12.4	26.0	44.4	14.5
Supervising the consumption of CDs on the pharmacy premises is an appropriate role for the community pharmacist	336	8.0	38.4	19.7	25.9	8.0
Collecting empty ampoules of prescribed opiates from the client is an appropriate role for the community pharmacist	338	5.0	30.5	27.8	29.0	7.7

relatively low incidence of injecting use in the region. As a result few services are currently offered by community pharmacists; however, it was encouraging to note that most appeared willing to offer services if required.

Community pharmacists have a clear role to play in many of the aims and objectives described in the *Drug Misuse in Northern Ireland; A Policy Statement* (Department of Health and Social Services, 1995) and in the *Drug Strategy for Northern Ireland* (Northern Ireland Drugs Campaign, 1999).

Pharmacists in Northern Ireland are already involved in health promotion activities, relating to alcohol use, smoking cessation, advice on diet and to a limited extent on drug misuse (e.g. through the distribution of information leaflets during national campaigns). With training, community pharmacists' health promotion role with respect to illicit drug use can be extended. With respect to treatment and rehabilitation, to date there has been little need for community pharmacy services; however, this will change with the commencement of needle exchange pilots in the region. Obviously, if the injecting drug problem escalates, there will be greater need for pharmacist contact with drug misusers, a role that they are willing to embrace. Pharmacists in the community could also play an important role in public education on drug misuse. In consideration of monitoring and evaluation, Sheridan *et al.*, (1996, 1997) concluded that pharmacists in England and Wales offered a network of contacts with drug misusers and as such were ideally placed to monitor patients for compliance. Such a role may evolve in Northern Ireland in the future.

Community pharmacists in Northern Ireland have some concerns regarding the provision of services for drug misusers. These include fear of violence or attack, reservations regarding the impact of drug misusers visiting their premises and concern regarding potential health risks posed to staff. Such concerns should be addressed with adequate training and the establishment of support systems. In addition, links should be established between pharmacists, prescribers and specialist services.

In summary, Northern Ireland is at an important stage in relation to illicit drug abuse, particularly intravenous misuse. Although the prevalence of misuse is relatively low at present, steps have already been taken to establish management policies. The policy makers and all organisations involved in this field in Northern Ireland have the luxury of hindsight, as the strengths and weakness of service provision in other parts of the UK and elsewhere can be taken into account during service development in Northern Ireland.

REFERENCES

Clinical Resource Efficiency Support Team (1999). *Northern Ireland protocol for opiate detoxification*, CREST, Belfast.

Craig J (1997). *Almost adult: Some correlates of alcohol, tobacco and illicit drug use among a sample of 16 and 17 year olds in Northern Ireland*, Northern Ireland Statistics and Research Agency, Belfast.

Department of Health and Social Services (Health Promotion Policy Branch) (1995). *Drug Misuse in Northern Ireland: a Policy Statement*, Department of Health and Social Services (Health Promotion Policy Branch), Belfast.

Health Promotion Agency for Northern Ireland (1995). *The health behaviour of school children in Northern Ireland: a report on the 1994 survey*, Health Promotion Agency for Northern Ireland, Belfast.

Health Promotion Agency for Northern Ireland (1996). *Illicit Drug Use in Northern Ireland: a handbook for professionals,* Health Promotion Agency for Northern Ireland, Belfast.

McEvoy K, McElrath K, Higgens K (1998). Does Ulster Still Say No? Drugs, politics and propaganda in Northern Ireland. *Journal of Drug Issues,* 28, 127–154.

Murray M (1994). Use of illegal drugs in Northern Ireland. In: Strang J and Gossop M (eds) *Heroin Addiction and Drug Policy: The British System.* Oxford University Press, Oxford. pp. 134–148.

Northern Ireland Drugs Campaign (1998). *Drugs in Northern Ireland: some key facts 1992–1998.* The Northern Ireland Office, Belfast.

Northern Ireland Drugs Campaign (1999). *Drug Strategy for Northern Ireland,* The Northern Ireland Office, Belfast.

Royal Ulster Constabulary (1995). *Chief Constable's Annual Report,* http://www.ruc. police.uk/report95/crime.htm

Sheridan J, Strang J, Barber N, Glanz A (1996). Role of community pharmacies in relation to HIV prevention and drug misuse: findings from the 1995 national survey in England and Wales. *British Medical Journal,* 313, 272–274.

Sheridan J, Strang J, Taylor C, Barber N (1997). HIV prevention and drug treatment services for drug misusers: a national study of community pharmacists' attitudes and their involvement in service specific training. *Addiction,* 92, 1737–1748.

Strang J, Sheridan J, Barber N (1996). Prescribing injectable and oral methadone to opiate addicts: Results from the 1995 national postal survey of community pharmacies in England and Wales. *British Medical Journal,* 313, 270–272.

7

The services provided by community pharmacists to prevent, minimise and manage drug misuse: an international perspective

Constantine Berbatis, V Bruce Sunderland and Max Bulsara

INTRODUCTION

This chapter reviews from an international perspective the services provided by community pharmacists to prevent, minimise and treat the harm of drug misuse. The services related to drug misuse will be reviewed, but with a focus on two in particular – the dispensing of pharmacotherapies for the management of drug dependence and the supply of clean injecting equipment for those who inject drugs. This division of services also serves as a reminder that many injectors inject drugs other than heroin (e.g. amphetamines, cocaine, steroids), and that not all those who inject drugs are drug dependent. Although the focus of this chapter may be mainly on opiate misuse, the focus on community pharmacy practice will be in the context of its involvement with a wide spectrum of drug misuse and those pharmacy services shown to be effective in preventing, minimising or treating drug misuse and its consequences.

Worldwide the prevalence of opioid dependence has grown enormously since 1970. Furthermore, the realisation in the 1980s of the importance of methadone programmes in preventing the transmission of HIV and hepatitis viruses (due to the sharing of needles and syringes by injecting drug users) has forced a major re-appraisal of practice as well as policy. Many countries have embraced harm minimisation policies and philosophies. The term refers to an approach which is "aimed at achieving intermediate goals as a half-way stage to achievement of the ultimate goal of freedom from drug dependence by using a variety of strategies to decrease the health and social risks and consequences of substance use..." (WHO, 1998). The main harm reduction interventions have been the provision of methadone treatment and needle/ syringe programmes which have been widely adapted through Europe, the United Kingdom, Australia and New Zealand (Wodak, 2000). The community-based treatment of opioid dependence has included GP prescribing and community pharmacy dispensing has grown in many parts of the world such as New Zealand, Europe, and Australia since the 1980s.

Community pharmacies in developed countries have many attributes that make them important in providing services to help prevent or manage drug misuse. For example, the geographical distribution of, and opening hours of pharmacies, make them accessible to the public for obtaining condoms (Pinkerton and Abramson, 1997), needles and syringes (Andreyev, 1985; Sheridan *et al.*, 2000) and daily dispensing of methadone (Muhleisen *et al.*, 1998), all of which are highly cost-effective with regard to minimising infections and other harms associated with drug misuse. The ability of pharmacists to dispense and supervise the consumption of methadone liquid on a daily basis enables them to complement specialist clinics not only to manage opiate dependence, but simultaneously to prevent the diversion of methadone (Scott *et al.*, 1994) and to reduce the spread of infections by injecting drug users. The high regard for pharmacists by the general public and their ready access to the public make them ideal for disseminating information on the prevention, minimisation, or management of drug misuse.

BACKGROUND TO THE EXTENT OF THE TREATMENT RESPONSE
By 2000, the number of people with opioid dependence being treated worldwide on a maintenance basis with opioid agonists or antagonists is probably:

- Over 500,000 people with oral methadone maintenance (Farrell and Hall, 1998)
- Over 60,000 with the partial agonist-antagonist oral buprenorphine including 55,000 in France (Obadia *et al.*, 2000)
- An estimated under 50 in approved clinical trials with oral controlled release morphine (Clark *et al.*, 2002)
- Over 1,000 with injectable morphine or heroin including 800 in Switzerland (Farrell and Hall, 1998)
- An estimated 3,000 opiate addicts in England who received injectable methadone (Sheridan *et al.*, 1996), but a much small number outside the UK
- An estimated over 1,000 receiving oral leva-alpha-acetylmethadol (LAAM) including 279 in the USA (Parrino, 2000).[1]

The international medical approach to opioid dependence however varies considerably. Whilst many countries have responded to the growing problem of opiate addiction by the provision of long-term methadone maintenance treatment, many other countries have no methadone available at all and have an alternative opiate maintenance programme using drugs such as those above. Other countries may have no opiate maintenance whatsoever, and rely solely on an abstinence-based model.

Whilst methadone is the most comprehensively researched and prescribed oral opiate substitute, other drugs such as buprenorphine are widely prescribed in countries such as France and India. In France, where instalments of more than one week are the norm after the induction phase, there have been concerns that the drug is being injected by a small proportion of patients, rather than being used sublingually, and that it is being diverted onto the illicit market (Picard, 1997).

---

[1] Due to adverse cardiac events, LAAM has been suspended in The European Union (EMEA, 2001).

Dihydrocodeine is also used in some countries such as the UK. In Germany, however, legislation has been brought in to control its prescription for opioid dependence due to concerns about codeine-related deaths (EMCDDA, 2000). Controlled-release morphine is being tested as an alternative therapy for opioid dependence (Wodak, 2001). Like methadone it has been reported to be highly diverted into self-injection in jurisdictions of Australia where heroin and/or methadone were in short supply. In these locations the misuse of controlled release forms of morphine approached rates of injecting use similar to those of illicit heroin (Berbatis *et al.*, 2000). It is important therefore for pharmacists who dispense these pharmacotherapies to be aware of their abuse potential and the patterns of licit and illicit drug misuse locally. This knowledge may be useful to share with prescribers and may assist to minimise the diversion of the controlled release forms of morphine into drug misuse.

THE INVOLVEMENT OF THE COMMUNITY PHARMACIST IN THE PROVISION OF PHARMACOTHERAPIES FOR THE MANAGEMENT OF OPIATE ADDICTION

The role of the community pharmacist in provision of treatment to opiate addicts varies greatly from one country to another. Nowadays, methadone occupies a dominant position amongst the opiate agonist pharmacotherapies. However, this has not always been so. In 1964 the first dependent heroin users were started on methadone treatment as inpatients in New York City hospitals and subsequently were treated in outpatient clinics and in other clinic programs (Ball and Ross, 1991). By December 1998, 785 methadone programmes (including 401 non-profit programmes) were licensed in the USA with 179,329 patients (Parrino, 2000). None of the methadone or other opioid pharmacotherapies however are dispensed by community pharmacists.

Clinic-based models for methadone treatment (Figure 7.1a) have subsequently been embraced and adapted in many countries up to the early 1980s. Several states in Australia, some European countries, New Zealand, the USA and recently Canada (Fischer, 2000) have developed systems which deliver methadone treatment by medical practitioners alone (Salsitz *et al.*, 2000) or with pharmacists in primary care settings (Muhleisen *et al.*, 1998).

The simplified structures of the main methadone programmes conducted in the USA are represented in Figures 7.1a and d. Other developed countries have, in addition, developed systems depicted in Figures 7.1b–e. In Europe, Australia and New Zealand the majority of patients in methadone programmes receive prescriptions from doctors which are then dispensed in community or primary care settings (Figures 7.1d and e) mainly in community pharmacies, but sometimes directly from a clinic. In France, however, the prescribing of methadone is limited to a small number of licensed doctors, and GPs tend to prescribe buprenorphine, the dispensing of which from community pharmacies has been approved since early 1996 (Moatti *et al.*, 1998). The community-based methadone programmes (Figure 7.1e) in Australia, New Zealand and parts of Europe usually involve doctors and pharmacies accredited by medical, pharmacy or state authorities to prescribe or dispense methadone (Muhleisen *et al.*, 1998), although currently such accreditation is not required either for pharmacists or doctors in the UK. By way of contrast, in the USA less than 1% of methadone patients are assessed and treated in community settings (Salsitz *et al.*, 2000; Parrino, 2000). Community-based methadone programmes in the USA involving the dispensing of

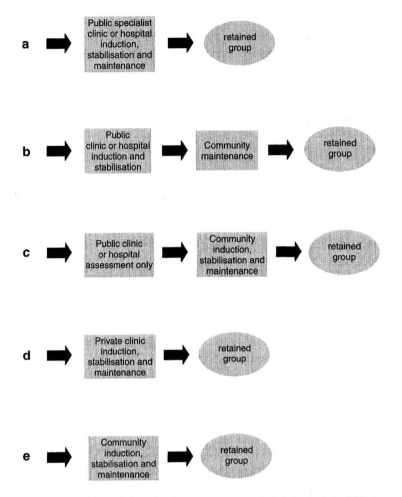

a: Hospital or specialist clinic-based methadone programmes typical of those in the USA &
   other countries e.g. UK
b: Hospital or specialist clinic based programmes typical of those in Australia (all states) and
   other countries e.g. UK
c: Joint hospital assessment and community programmes (e.g. Australian Capital Territory, UK)
d: Private clinic-based programmes typical of those in USA and Australia
e: Community-based programmes typical of those in UK, Europe, Australia, and New Zealand.

Figure 7.1 Methadone programmes: different structures.

methadone in community pharmacies started on a trial basis in 2001 in New York City.
Where the treatment of opioid dependence in primary care is the norm, pharmacy educators and regulatory bodies should ensure undergraduate teaching, appropriate training, and continuing education programmes are instituted for the profession.

In Europe, the proportion of opiate users in the population varies. For example,
Germany, Finland, Denmark, Ireland, France, Greece, Sweden, the Netherlands and
Belgium have an estimated 200–400 problem opiate users per 100,000 population
aged 15–64, whilst in Portugal, Spain and the UK it is estimated to be 400–600 per
100,000 population aged 24–60, and in Italy and Luxembourg over 600 per 100,000

population aged 24–60 (EMCDDA, 2000). Table 7.1, adapted from *EMCDDA Insights, No. 3* (EMCDDA, 2000) gives details of the types of drugs prescribed, treatments available and involvement of community pharmacists in service provision. These data clearly show treatment varies within the European Union. For example treatment in Greece is mainly based on an abstinence model, with up to 70% of treatment being for detoxification, whereas in France, Ireland, Sweden and Portugal, treatment is mainly maintenance based. However, even within these four countries the range of pharmacotherapies varies, with Sweden and Ireland only prescribing methadone, whilst Portugal also uses LAAM and France primarily uses buprenorphine (doctors need to be licensed to prescribe methadone but not buprenorphine).

The activities of pharmacists varies considerably across different European countries. For example, in the UK and Luxembourg, pharmacists are involved in dispensing pharmacotherapies whilst Greece does not permit pharmacy dispensing. In Germany, with the exception of Hamburg, methadone is mainly dispensed by GPs in their surgeries. In Italy, pharmacists are able to sell naloxone (the opioid antagonist used to reverse opioid overdose) without the need for a prescription.

In some countries pharmacists supervise the consumption of drugs such as methadone in the pharmacy. Supervised consumption guarantees compliance with treatment and minimises diversion. In Scotland community pharmacists in Glasgow supervise the consumption of 76% of the dispensed doses of methadone (Roberts and Bryson, 1999). Supervision is widely available in Australia and New Zealand and in parts of England, Wales, and Ireland.

On the other side of the world, in Australia, methadone treatment was first prescribed for opioid dependence by community clinicians and dispensed by community pharmacists in 1969. By 1972, pharmacists in Victoria's Austin Hospital became the first involved in a comprehensive hospital inpatient methadone programme (Berbatis, 1998; Hynes, 1975). The number of dependent heroin users in Australia more than doubled over a decade, from an estimated 34,000 in 1984–1987 to 74,000 in 1997 (Hall *et al.*, 2000). From 1969 the national total on methadone treatment grew to approximately 5,000 in 1986, to nearly 25,000 by 1998 (Berbatis *et al*, 2000) and 32,000 by 2000, ranking second pro rata in the world after Switzerland (Berbatis *et al.*, 2000). In New South Wales which has the highest per capita use of methadone liquid in the world (Berbatis *et al*, 2000), methadone clinics, using nurse dispensing to cope with the high demand for services, have been operational since the 1980s and in 2000 the majority of methadone was still dispensed from them. In Australia this development has involved the continuous active recruitment and training of community medical practitioners and community pharmacists in all states, as well as specialist and public hospital clinics. Incentives for recruiting pharmacists to methadone programmes were shown to be effective in the Australian Capital Territory and Tasmania (Berbatis and Sunderland, 2000).

The fear of a high risk of violent property crimes against methadone pharmacies has been cited as inhibiting pharmacies from joining methadone programmes (Advisory Council on the Misuse of Drugs, 1993). An analysis made of insurance claims submitted by non-methadone and methadone pharmacies from two states in Australia over the period 1996–2000 found no significant difference (Berbatis and Sunderland, 2000). This supported an earlier negative finding from a comparison of reported property crimes from pharmacies in one state. Increasing the participation

Table 7.1 Comparisons of treatment availability and pharmacy involvement in the European Union. (Adapted from information in EMCDDA 2000)

Country	Methadone treatment available from	Other substitution treatments	Maintenance or detoxification	Community pharmacy involvement
Belgium	1997	None	No information	No information available
Denmark	1970	LAAM and buprenorphine (1998)	50–75% aimed at maintenance	Limited pharmacy dispensing. Until 1996 gave free needles and syringes
Germany	1992	Buprenorphine (2000)	50–75% aimed at maintenance	Methadone may be dispensed since 1998 (in Hamburg since 1988). Only minor role in needle exchange
Greece	1993	None	Primarily detox (<30% aimed at maintenance)	Pharmacies not permitted to dispense methadone
Spain	1983	LAAM (1997)	50–75% aimed at maintenance	Methadone may be dispensed since 1996, but few do so. More pharmacies involved in needle exchange. Both services have been encouraged
France	1995	Buprenorphine (1996)	75–100% aimed at maintenance	Pharmacies can dispense methadone, Subutex, morphine and codeine sulphate. Also involved in needle exchange
Ireland	1992	None	75–100% aimed at maintenance	Dispense methadone including supervising consumption on-site
Italy	1975	Buprenorphine (1996)	Primarily detox (<30% aimed at maintenance)	Sell injecting equipment, and can sell naloxone to heroin users without a prescription

Luxembourg	1989	Mephenon® (1989) buprenorphine (2000)	No information	Can dispense methadone and sell syringes
Netherlands	1968	Heroin (1997)	50–75% aimed at maintenance	Can dispense methadone (no further information available)
Austria	1987	Buprenorphine (1997) and slow-release morphine (1998)	50–75% aimed at maintenance	Dispense opioid substitution therapy under supervision
Portugal	1977	LAAM (1994)	75–100% aimed at maintenance	Since 1993, all pharmacies have started to offer needle exchange Currently 2000 providing service. Pilot service for substitution dispensing currently underway
Finland	1974	Buprenorphine (1997)	50–75% aimed at maintenance	No information available
Sweden	1967	None	75–100% aimed at maintenance	No information available
United Kingdom	1968	Buprenorphine (1999) Heroin	50–75% aimed at maintenance	Pharmacies can dispense methadone (sometimes under supervision), sell syringes and provide them free in needle exchange schemes

rate of community pharmacies in methadone programmes improves access for opioid dependants into methadone programmes and complements dosing in clinics where the congregation of opioid dependants creates a poor milieu. Community pharmacies improve the flexibility and convenience of dosing for patients. Transfers of methadone patients from other programmes and dosing are as convenient as in clinics (Muhleisen *et al.*, 1998; Gill, 1999). Finally, significantly higher retention of methadone patients was recently found in community-based methadone programmes with pharmacists providing daily supervised consumption of methadone compared with patients in public specialist clinics in Australia (Berbatis & Sunderland, 2000). The results consistently show the benefits of community-based methadone programmes and particularly where methadone consumption is supervised in pharmacies.

THE PROVISION OF STERILE INJECTING EQUIPMENT

In addition to the dispensing of pharmacotherapies, the other main area of involvement of community pharmacists in services for drug misusers is the supply of clean injecting equipment either by sale or needle exchange. Although many countries have now adopted pharmacy-based needle exchange schemes, this has not always been the case. In early 1982 in the UK, pharmacists were advised by their professional body that they should not supply drug users with syringes (RPSGB, 1982), further stigmatising drug users. However, with the threat of HIV, this ruling was overturned allowing pharmacists to sell needles and syringes to injecting drug users and paving the way for needle exchange services, with a move from the pharmacist simply being a supplier of equipment to being someone who both delivered clean equipment and collected used equipment.

The involvement of pharmacists in the supply of injecting equipment, like their involvement in dispensing, differs from country to country. For example in England, Wales and Scotland pharmacists can offer free needle exchange services – both the supply and collection of equipment being funded by the government, whilst in New Zealand, drug users must pay for their equipment. In Australia, over 500 pharmacies in New South Wales participate in the Fitpack Scheme which provides 1 ml syringes for purchase and many pharmacies exchange them free on return of a pack of used syringes. Over 50% of community pharmacies in Australia offer sterile injecting equipment either by sale or through an exchange programme to the estimated 100,000–175,000 regular or occasional injecting drug users. In France, whilst pharmacists can supply needles and syringes through needle exchange, they tend to do so by supplying vouchers which can be inserted into a needle exchange machine which is attached to the outside of the pharmacy premises.

OTHER PHARMACY SERVICES

In 2000, 1,557 or 31% of Australia's nearly 5,000 registered public and private pharmacies were approved to provide methadone treatment although up to one-fifth of these may be inactive at any given time (Berbatis and Sunderland, 2000). Approved "methadone" pharmacies typically employ pharmacists who are additionally trained and accredited. They monitor prescriptions for other concurrent dependence-producing or potentially interacting drugs. Pharmacists also assess patients prior to dosing for adverse signs of alcohol or other agents affecting behaviour and to monitor the responses to methadone treatment to assess the effectiveness (or adequacy of dose), or toxicity (excessive dose) of methadone. One study of Victoria's methadone pharmacists found a disturbing 32% who would dispense methadone to an intoxicated patient (Koutroulis *et al.*, 2000).

In Western Australia, the Australian Pharmacy Foundation was established in June 2000 to broaden the role of pharmacists in the prevention of drug misuse in the community. It is funded by a government grant and donations from the sales of "Fitpacks" (needle and syringe packs) through pharmacies (Lenton *et al.*, 2000). In June 2000 it implemented a project to reduce drug overdose deaths. The "Drug Aware" project, also in Western Australia, promotes the provision of drug and alcohol information through community pharmacies.

Pharmacists involved in methadone programmes in Switzerland (Swiss Narcotics Commission, 1996), and some methadone pharmacies in the Australian Capital Territory arrange urinalyses ordered by methadone prescribers. The degree of involvement by pharmacists varies. They may simply prompt methadone patients of the time they are required to provide specimens to the designated laboratories, or provide containers to patients for their urine specimens to be analysed by laboratories, or receive the urinalysis results to discuss with methadone prescribers for the purpose of guiding further treatment (Berbatis, 1999).

Condoms have been available from pharmacies since the 1920s and their reliability has improved markedly. They lower the probability of sexually transmitted HIV by at least 90% and they are effective against bacterial sexually transmitted diseases at very low cost (Pinkerton and Abramson, 1997).

During the twentieth century community pharmacists in most developed countries were made legally responsible for maintaining detailed records of medically prescribed opioids and amphetamines. From these data patients, prescribers, dispensers and stocks maintained can be identified. Drug use can be therefore monitored by government agencies, professional and other bodies. In turn, these individual drug use data complement overall national and jurisdictional or regional statistics held by most countries. This allows them to compare trends of licit drugs between jurisdictions within countries or between nations, hence identifying locations with high questionable use which may be investigated and acted upon (Berbatis *et al.*, 2000).

Other more specialised services exist such as the, "Pharmacists Against Substance Abuse", in Jamaica. Members of this group are trained in counselling techniques and offer basic counselling and referral and pharmacies act as data gathering centres for the National Council on Drug Abuse (Campbell-Grizzle, 2000). Although the main drug of misuse is cannabis and not opiates, pharmacies are able to make an impact on the health of these clients.

In the UK a small pilot study indicated that drug users' dental health was significantly poorer than that of an age and gender matched population (Sheridan *et al.*, 2001).

CONCLUSIONS

Community pharmacies can offer less costly and more effective alternatives to clinics as providers of methadone and other pharmacotherapies, and appear to be more effective in retaining patients on methadone treatment and reducing the rate of diversion of methadone onto the illicit market. Essential to minimising the risks of methadone toxicity and enhancing effectiveness is an improved clinical skill in assessing the medication history of methadone patients prior to dispensing, and monitoring the effects of treatment in-patients. Frequent communication with prescribers is recommended during the commencement or induction of patients on methadone treatment. Supervised administration is crucial in enhancing the effectiveness of methadone by increasing compliance and significantly improving retention, while lowering the risk of diversion.

The involvement of pharmacies in offering public health services such as providing ready access to condoms and to sterile needles is very important because of the outstanding cost-benefits to society. For example, the efficiency of needle and syringe programmes in the prevention of infection and deaths caused by HIV and the savings to health care systems are so large that community pharmacy's participation in both needle exchange and supply programmes should become widely adopted throughout the world.

REFERENCES

Advisory Council on the Misuse of Drugs (1993). *AIDS and drug misuse update*, HMSO, London.
Andreyev HJ (1985). Selling syringes to drug addicts. *Lancet*, 2, 1192–1193.
Ball JC, Ross A (1991). *The effectiveness of methadone maintenance treatment: patients, programs, services and outcome*, Springer-Verlag, New York.
Berbatis C (1999). *Pharmacists in methadone maintenance or opioid replacement programs for the treatment of opiate dependence*, School of Pharmacy, Curtin University, Perth, p. 17.
Berbatis CG (1998). Methadone programs, harm reduction, chronic diseases and hospital pharmacists. *Australian Journal of Hospital Pharmacy*, 28, 41–44.
Berbatis CG, Sunderland VB (2000). *The role of community pharmacy in methadone maintenance treatment. Final report*, Australian Association of Consultant Pharmacy, Barton (ACT).
Berbatis CG, Sunderland VB, Bulsara M, Lintzeris N (2000). Trends in licit opioid use in Australia, 1984–1998: comparative analysis of international and jurisdictional data. *Medical Journal of Australia*, 173, 524–527.
Campbell Grizzle E (2000). Pharmacists Against Substance Abuse (PASA) – The Jamaican model. *PharMAGazine*, 3(10), 1–2.
Clark N, Khoo K, Lintzeis N, Ritter A, Whelan G (2002). A randomized trial of once-daily slow-release oral morphine versus methadone for heroin dependence. *Drug and Alcohol Dependence*, 66, s33.
EMCDDA (2000). *Insights No 3: Reviewing current practice in drug-substitution treatment in the European Union*, EMCDDA, Luxembourg.
EMEA (2001). EMEA public statement on the recommendation to suspend The marketing authorisation for Orlaam (levacetylmethadol) in the European Union, 19/4/2001. URL: http://www.emea.eu.int
Farrell M, Hall W (1998). The Swiss heroin trials: testing alternative approaches. *British Medical Journal*, 316, 639.
Fischer B (2000). Prescriptions, power and politics: the turbulent history of methadone maintenance in Canada. *Journal of Public Health Policy*, 21, 187–209.
Gill T (1999). *The New South Wales methadone maintenance treatment: clinical practice guidelines*, North Sydney, NSW Health Department.
Hall WD, Ross JE, Lynskey MT, Law MG, Degenhardt LJ (2000). How many dependent heroin users are there in Australia? *Medical Journal of Australia*, 173, 528–531.

Hynes K (1975). The role of the hospital pharmacist in methadone treatment. *Australian Journal of Hospital Pharmacy*, 5, 27–31.

Koutroulis GY, Kutin JJ, Ugoni AM, Odgers P, Muhleisen P, Ezard N, Lintzeris N, Stowe A, Lanagan A (2000). Pharmacists' provision of methadone to intoxicated clients in community pharmacies, Victoria, Australia. *Drug and Alcohol Review*, 19, 299–308.

Lenton S, Kerry K, Loxley W, Tan-Quigley A, Greig R (2000). Citizens who inject drugs: the 'Fitpack study'. *International Journal of Drug Policy*, 11, 285–297.

Moatti JP, Souville M, Escaffre N, Obadia Y (1998). French General Practitioners' Attitudes Toward Maintenance Drug Abuse Treatment With Buprenorphine. *Addiction*, 93, 1567–1575.

Muhleisen P, Lintzeris N, Koutroulis G, Odgers P, Stowe A, Lanagan A, Ezard N (1998). Evaluation of methadone dispensing in community pharmacies in Victoria. *Australian Pharmacist Supplement*, 17(8), 7–12.

Obadia Y, Perrin V, Feroni I, Vlahov D, Moatti JP (2000). Injecting misuse of buprenorphine among French drug users. *Addiction*, 96, 267–272.

Parrino M (2000). American Methadone Treatment Association, 217 Broadway Street, Suite 304, New York NY, 10007. Personal communication, December 2000.

Picard G (1997). Current use of buprenorphine in France: a pharmacists' survey. *Research and Clinical Forums*, 19, 33–40.

Pinkerton SD, Abramson PR (1997). Condoms and the prevention of AIDS. *American Scientist*, 85, 364–373.

Roberts K, Bryson S (1999). The contribution of Glasgow pharmacists to the management of drug misuse. *Hospital Pharmacist*, 6, 244–248.

Royal Pharamaceutical Socity Great Britain (1982). Sale of syringes. *Pharmaceutical Journal*, 228, 692.

Salsitz EA, Joseph H, Frank B, Perez J, Richman BL, Salomon N, Kalin MF, Novick DM (2000). Methadone medical maintenance (MMM): treating chronic opioid dependence in private medical practice – a summary report (1983–1998). *Mount Sinai Journal of Medicine*, 67, 388–397.

Scott RT, Burnett SJ, McNutty H (1994). Supervised administration of methadone by pharmacists. *British Medical Journal*, 308, 1438.

Sheridan J, Aggleton M, Carson T (2001). Dental health and access to dental treatment: a comparison of drug users and non-drug users attending community pharmacies. *British Dental Journal*, 191, 453–457.

Sheridan J, Lovell S, Parsons J, Turnbull J, Stimson GV, Strang J (2000). Pharmacy-based needle exchange (PBNX) schemes in South-East London. *Addiction*, 95, 1551–1560.

Sheridan J, Strang J, Barber N, Glanz A (1996). Role of community pharmacies in relation to HIV prevention and drug misuse: findings from the 1995 national survey in England and Wales. *British Medical Journal*, 313, 272–274.

Swiss Narcotics Commission (1996). *Swiss methadone report: narcotic substitution in the treatment of heroin addicts in Switzerland*, Third edition. Swiss Federal Office of Public Health and Addiction Research Foundation, Berne. 67–72.

WHO Expert Committee on Drug Dependence (1998). *WHO technical report series 873. Treatment of drug dependence*, World Health Organisation, Geneva.

Wodak A (2000). Developing more effective responses to illicit drugs in Australia. In: *Heroin crisis*, Bookman, Melbourne. 197–210.

Wodak A (2001). Drug treatment for opioid dependence. *Australian Prescriber*, 24, 4–7.

8

Drug users and pharmacists: the clients' perspective

Catriona Matheson

INTRODUCTION

Taking the client's perspective into account is essential when delivering a relevant and user-friendly service. This chapter considers the drug user's perspective of community pharmacy services. It is based on unpublished and published research conducted in Scotland (Matheson, 1998a–c; Neale, 1998a,b, 1999) the author having been part of this research team, and published research conducted in London (Sheridan and Barber, 1996). These studies specifically covered the client's perspective of pharmacy services.

In the Scottish study interviews were conducted with 124 drug users to gain their in-depth views and experiences of community pharmacies. Interviewees were selected from a sample of 23 pharmacies and eight drug agencies in the four main Scottish cities (Aberdeen, Dundee, Edinburgh and Glasgow) and their adjacent rural areas. The pharmacies were identified from previous research as having involvement with drug users. Two researchers (Matheson and Neale) conducted 40 and 84 interviews respectively using identical topic guides.

The factors which affect a drug user's choice of a pharmacy are described, including what they think about the availability of services such as substitute prescribing, the supervised self-administration of methadone, selling or exchanging injecting equipment and health advice or information services. In addition the process of service delivery is considered, for example their opinions of how they are treated, and what they think about the level of privacy in pharmacies.

DRUG USERS' VIEWS OF PHARMACY SERVICES
Choice of pharmacy

Why does a drug user choose a particular pharmacy? Is it primarily for reasons of privacy or anonymity? Given that drug users could be subject to stigmatisation they may feel particularly sensitive to using a pharmacy in which they feel they stand out from the rest of the customers/clients. However, data from drug users did not generally show this to be the case. In fact a drug user often chooses a pharmacy mainly for geographical convenience, either because it is close to home or perhaps because it is near other amenities such as schools and shops. In this respect, drug users probably do not differ from other pharmacy clients. However, for some drug users their choice was affected by how they were treated in a previous pharmacy, and the perceived attitude of the pharmacist and/or staff, a theme which is further explored later in this chapter.

Other factors were also important. For some clients the attitude of the pharmacist was less important than the brand of methadone dispensed in a particular pharmacy. The opening hours of pharmacies were important to some drug users particularly those who work and need a pharmacy that opens late. For a few clients the level of anonymity was important in their choice of pharmacy. In addition, drug users may not want to be known or recognised by other drug users as the following interview quote demonstrated:

> *"There's a lot of people hanging around the one at [place name] an' I don't really want to be known, I suppose".*

Other factors which affected choice of pharmacy for some individuals were: the availability of certain services; the avoidance of other people; being barred from elsewhere; a pharmacy had been recommended by someone; a desire to reserve one pharmacy for a prescription and another pharmacy for injecting equipment due to a fear of jeopardising their prescription.

Provision of needles and syringes

In the UK clean injecting equipment can be distributed either through a needle/syringe exchange scheme (either stand alone, linked to a drug agency or pharmacy-based) or by sale through community pharmacies. Both systems have legal restrictions. In the needle/syringe scheme in Scotland if the client returned used equipment they could receive up to 15 clean sets of equipment, however if they do not return equipment they could only receive a maximum of five sets of equipment. This is based on guidance from the Lord Advocate in Scotland. In the rest of the UK no such restrictions apply. Pharmacists selling injecting equipment often supply insulin syringes which come in 1ml or 0.5ml sizes only. However, in some parts of the UK, e.g. the south-east of England, other sizes of syringes are available in pharmacies (Sheridan *et al.*, 2000). It is at the pharmacist's discretion whether or not they decide to sell equipment. If they do provide needles through sale or exchange they are recommended by the Pharmaceutical Society's Code of Ethics to have a sharps container or "cin-bin" on site. A "cin-bin" is a tough plastic bin used for the safe disposal of injecting equipment. "Cin-bins" are collected routinely for incineration (from which the name derives).

Neale analysed the clients' perspective of the provision of injecting equipment for the whole sample of 124 drug users previously described. Unless otherwise stated, this section draws from these findings (Neale, 1998a). Many drug users felt that the current availability of sterile injecting equipment was insufficient to meet demand and additional provision was required. Drug users argued that there should be at least one local source of sterile equipment in each area. Others stressed the need for outlets to be open for longer hours, especially in the evenings and at weekends. Indeed, where sterile equipment was not on hand, many believed that drug users still shared equipment as this interview quote indicates:

> *"There is not enough places for them and people are still using needles, sharing them".*

Drug users often had very little information about which local pharmacies provided needles, sterile swabs and personal sharps containers. Likewise, many drug users did not know which pharmacies accepted returned needles and some drug users may not have even realised that such a service existed. Pharmacists were not perceived by clients as being very systematic about collecting returned needles, even where an official exchange was operating.

A need for more publicity regarding which pharmacies were providing a needle service and at what times was highlighted by drug users. Some drug agencies have leaflets and posters explaining which local pharmacies provided needle services in the region. However, many users do not attend these agencies and hence they do not see this information. For those visiting unfamiliar areas, this lack of knowledge could be particularly problematic.

Embarrassment was a major factor determining how drug users both accessed and disposed of their injecting equipment. Both Sheridan and Barber (1996) and Neale (1998a) discussed how some drug users felt that it was not difficult to enter a pharmacy and ask for needles, while others found it extremely awkward or even degrading. Some clients felt able to obtain needles from the pharmacy where they obtained their prescription for oral methadone, but others felt that this was not possible because the pharmacist would not allow it or because they were personally too embarrassed. Some injectors preferred to frequent a pharmacy where they were known so that they did not have to explain what they wanted. Others simply asked friends to collect or dispose of equipment on their behalf as this quote illustrates:

"Mostly [the drug agency exchange] eh my boyfriend would go down and they would give us..."

Since many clients may be uncomfortable about going into unfamiliar surroundings to ask whether injecting equipment was available or could be returned, well-publicised discreet and friendly services could attract drug users from further afield. Conversely, an unfriendly or hostile agency could deter individuals from ever returning, regardless of how nearby it was as the following quote from Neale's (1998a) paper demonstrates.

"As I say, I wouldn't even ask for needles in here. I wouldn't give them [the pharmacy staff] the satisfaction. As I say, I go to certain places".

Pharmacies were considered the most accessible sources of clean injecting equipment, although they tended only to provide a limited range of services. Centralised needle exchanges had more specialist staff and offered more services (advice, health care, leaflets and family planning), but were less convenient in terms of location and opening hours. Centralised agencies also posed problems for individuals who wanted to avoid other drug users or who did not have the money to travel across town. Additionally, some drug users felt that needle/syringe exchanges were less useful for casual users who might have nothing to exchange or who might only want a single syringe.

Regardless of outlet type, however, most drug users felt that injecting equipment should be free rather than sold since users often did not have any money. Likewise, most drug users agreed that it was better to provide equipment on an exchange basis (and with a compulsory personal "cin-bin") rather than to give them away without any provision for their safe disposal. It was also generally believed that any form of availability was better than nothing and ultimately more outlets rather than less were required in order to stop the spread of diseases such as hepatitis and HIV.

Prescribed methadone

Neale also analysed drug users' views of prescribed methadone (Neale, 1998b). This section draws on these findings unless otherwise stated.

Methadone was described by drug users as a complex drug with multiple advantages, but simultaneously causing many problems for those receiving it. At one extreme, methadone was considered a life-saver and at the other extreme a dangerous drug which should be taken off the market. Few felt that prescribed methadone had no negative effects for drug users and very few drug users argued that it had no benefits at all. Most clients had mixed views about whether methadone was helpful or unhelpful as the following interview quote from Neale's paper illustrated.

"Methadone gives you a lot of problems and it takes a lot of your problems away".

The main reported benefits of methadone were that it helped people to stop using drugs, prevented withdrawals, stopped people injecting and prevented crime. Additionally, methadone enabled drug users to cope with their problems, to feel in control and to regain some self-respect and confidence. Methadone allowed drug users to feel normal and helped them to lead a normal lifestyle. Some drug users felt that a methadone prescription increased their energy, time, and money. As a result, personal relationships were improved because they no longer needed to spend the entire day trying to obtain drugs. Consequently they also had the energy and the time to think about and do other things, such as spending time with their children or seeking paid employment.

The main negative things said about methadone were that it was very addictive and it was often abused. Methadone could be seen as replacing one addiction with another or perhaps even starting an addiction. Many drug users believed that methadone was responsible for causing similar or worse problems than heroin and other street drugs, as this interview quote demonstrated.

"The withdrawals are far, far worse than heroin or anything else. Its the worst I've ever experienced".

Many drug users complained that methadone caused lethargy, aching joints, dental decay, weight loss or weight gain. Additionally, some believed that prescribed methadone had resulted in the deaths of some drug users and caused personality changes in others.

Overall, most drug users would not describe methadone as entirely beneficial or completely harmful and it would therefore be inaccurate to claim that they tend to be either "for" or "against" its use as a substitute drug. Indeed, many drug users recognised that the value of methadone for any given individual depended on the particular circumstances of that individual in time, rather than the particular dosage of methadone.

Dispensing and supervised self-administration of methadone

This section is mainly based on findings from Sheridan and Barber (1996) and Neale (1998c).

Pharmacists dispense a range of drugs for the management of drug misuse but the most common drug dispensed in the UK is methadone. In 1995, 96% of all opiate prescriptions (n = 3846) from a survey of one in four community pharmacies in England and Wales were for methadone (Strang *et al.*, 1996). Similarly in Scotland in 1995 a cross sectional survey of all community pharmacies revealed 3387 methadone prescriptions (Matheson *et al.*, 1999). By 2001 this had increased 2.6 fold (Matheson *et al.*, in press) Other drugs provided include benzodiazepines, dihydrocodeine, injectable diamorphine and other opiates. These drug may be dispensed in the same way as any other prescription but in practice often cover shorter time periods e.g. a week or a fortnight rather than one or two months. Pharmacists are bound by their NHS contract to dispense drugs on an NHS prescription and so they cannot refuse to dispense a prescription. In Scotland there is far less variation in the range of drugs prescribed and therefore dispensed and the great majority of prescriptions are for methadone (see Chapter 5). Another difference between Scotland and the rest of the UK is the proportion of methadone which is consumed on the pharmacy premises by the client under the pharmacist's supervision. This is called supervised administration of methadone (SAM) or supervised self-administration of methadone (SSAM) and this is covered in more detail in Chapter 12.

Although many drug users believed that supervised methadone consumption prevented abuse of the prescribing system and was therefore a good thing, many individuals felt that supervision was degrading and unfair. Some drug users were indifferent to supervision (sometimes qualifying this with "as long as it is private" or "as long as the shop is empty"); others felt that they had needed supervision initially but not as treatment continued.

From the clients' perspective the main advantage of supervision was that it prevented abuse of the system (that is individuals selling, exchanging, "topping up", or giving away their prescription). Additionally, there is some recognition that supervision assisted some individuals in sticking to the programme and protected others from the dangers of illicit drug use, particularly overdose and injecting. Supervised consumption was also proof that one was actually taking the full dosage. Moreover, for those desperate for their medication, consumption in the pharmacy provided a safe place for the immediate relief of painful withdrawals.

Supervision was mainly disliked because users found it embarrassing, degrading and stigmatising, as the following interview quote illustrated:

> "For Joe Public to see it, I think it's disgusting ... ah mean your prescription should be a private thing ... it's more a kick in the teeth to the person who's prescribed it. It's like takin' them down a wee bit".

This theme is further explored later in this chapter.

Use of pharmacies for advice and information services

When asking clients about whether they ever looked at leaflets in the pharmacy, whether on drug-related topics or on more general health issues, interest varied from those with a great desire for knowledge on any health-related matter to those who simply were not interested. A few drug users expressed a great desire for knowledge and would pick up leaflets on anything. Such individuals also often mentioned that they referred to books or went to the library, further indicating their need for information. However, many clients never looked at leaflets from the pharmacy, often because they were not interested. However, it may also be due to inherent limitations of this form of information-giving, such as having difficulty concentrating as the following interview quote demonstrates:

"I canna concentrate when I am trying to read because of my mental illness".

Generally leaflets related to drug misuse were welcomed and, in interviews, clients gave specific topics which they believed would be useful, such as an accurate account of how a person feels when undergoing detoxification, information on specific drugs and information on how methadone actually made a person feel (a user's perspective).

Some drug users never looked at drug-related leaflets in the pharmacy perhaps because they felt they knew enough already or because they had information from other sources such as drug agencies.

"Well to tell you the truth I've never really noticed about that like, not so much in the chemist, I would image that they do have leaflets I've just never really looked but you get leaflets and all that up at the [drug agency]".

Other barriers existed such as not wanting to be seen to be interested in a sensitive topic such as HIV.

Many drug users had asked the pharmacists for general health advice and advice was often sought regarding their children's health. Drug users do not differ from other members of the public in this respect. Similar to other members of the public they would ask for advice on a range of health problems for example, sore throats, cold sores, constipation, menstrual problems etc. These clients generally viewed the pharmacist as approachable and sympathetic. The pharmacist could be seen as a sounding board whom they consulted before the general practitioner to perhaps seek the pharmacist's opinion about whether they should go to the general practitioner. In such instances the pharmacist was seen as easier and more convenient than the general practitioner, particularly if the drug user felt they did not like to bother the general practitioner.

"Well we do ask him [the pharmacist] if there is something wrong wi the weans [children] if we don't think it is serious enough to go to the doctor".

Fewer clients approached a pharmacist as a source of advice/information on illicit drugs or drugs prescribed for drug misuse compared to advice on general health issues. The queries that were made tended to relate to injecting equipment or to the identification of illicit drugs. However, on occasion a pharmacist had provided advice to encourage an injecting drug user to seek treatment as this quote from an interview illustrates:

"I've known him for years but I've only been gettin' ma methadone off him for about 8 month out here. I've known him for a long time. It wis him that said to me you should get on methadone cos ma boyfriend's been goin' there for 2 year, he wis one o' the first ones that got it oot there. An' it wis him that recommended us".

Many clients would not ask a pharmacist for advice regarding illicit drugs. There was a fear that the pharmacist would disapprove or they feel their drug use was a private matter. There seemed to be a conflict between what is an illegitimate action (i.e. illicit drug use) and seeking advice from a legitimate, professional source. As the following quote illustrated:

> *"I think they would probably disapprove [the pharmacist]. I think they would know all about it, I just don't fancy asking a chemist about it. No if you're going into that sort of stuff you should at least know what you're doing with it, you shouldn't be asking the chemist to help you out".*

Very few drug users had experienced pharmacists discussing safe disposal of injecting equipment with their drug-using customers. To what extent users believed pharmacists should provide such advice was, however, a debatable point. An open shop may not have been considered a suitable location for such discussions or some drug using customers were not believed to be receptive to advice, or perhaps pharmacists were considered to be too busy or not having the appropriate expertise. Some drug users believed that injectors already knew about safe disposal or that information relating to injecting was better provided by specialist drug agencies, counsellors, other drug users or leaflets. In contrast, others felt that pharmacists should always discuss injection-related topics and should always remind users to dispose of equipment carefully.

Whilst seeking advice from pharmacists on illicit drug use is controversial, seeking advice on drugs prescribed for a drug problem was perhaps seen as more acceptable and more widely practised. The following example illustrates the sort of advice sought by clients:

> *"I was saying to [pharmacist's name] a few weeks ago, I says '[pharmacist's name] your going to sleep with that methadone and I canny sleep with it' ..... it's like an amphetamine, well to me it is, ... and [pharmacist's name] says 'well keep your diazepam for at night".*

In instances where advice was sought from a pharmacist, whether on general health, prescribed drugs or illicit drugs it appeared to be valued and taken seriously.

CLIENT INTERACTION WITH PHARMACISTS AND PHARMACY STAFF
The stigma of illicit drug use
In general drug users felt stigmatised. Use of a pharmacy in relation to their drug use was seen as aggravating that stigma, because of the visibility of requesting injecting equipment, consuming methadone on the premises and even collecting prescriptions to take away. Whilst some of these indicators would only be evident to the pharmacist and/or staff and not to the general public, the drug user still felt self-conscious and concerned about what others might think or say (Matheson, 1998a).

Drug users themselves had prejudices against particular types of behaviour in drug use, and differentiated between what is acceptable to them and what is not. Drug users' own prejudices were relevant to how they viewed prejudice directed at themselves from other people. The most obvious example of this was the view that oral ingestion or smoking of drugs was more acceptable than injecting:

> *"I think the sort of taboo about heroin came down a wee bit. I mean I certainly had a thing about never touching heroin and junkies and that but when you actually try, it kind of dispels those images cos you're smoking it which kind of makes you think it's OK".*

Drug users' own terminology gave strong indications of their views. Generally "junkie" was a term used to described the "worst" type of drug user and was usually associated with injecting. Drug users may often consider themselves to be "drug users", or "drug addicts" but not "junkies". Such individuals may look down on people who they considered to be "junkies". The word "junkie" also seemed to be associated with a particular visual image of a drug user – i.e. a pale, ill, unwashed, rather downtrodden individual.

Some believed that pharmacists (and the wider public in general), automatically associated drug use with HIV and AIDS, which in turn are associated with injecting behaviour.

> "...they think 'cause you're on medication that your a junky ken [you know], virus and AIDS and ignorance".

Clients felt they were immediately labelled according to their prescription and were then treated according to the pharmacist's view of the stereotypical drug user, which appeared to be akin to the drug user's view of a "junkie". Some believed that the pharmacist would assume the worst of them as a result of the stereotyping of drug users e.g. assuming they would shoplift.

The behaviour of pharmacists and drug users

The way a pharmacist handled a drug user could affect the way the drug user behaved and conversely the behaviour of the drug user could affect the handling by the pharmacist (Matheson, 1998b). The stigma associated with illicit drug use is a major factor in both how the user perceives they are handled by pharmacists and how they react. If a client has a very poor self-image which was subsequently reinforced by what they perceive to be negative handling in the pharmacy, they may be more likely to react negatively by shoplifting, being rude or even aggressive.

> "it would be different if it was sort of [pharmacy name] and things like that lowering their nose at you so like you lower them even more so like you maybe steal from them and laugh at them..."

As we have already seen, the drug users' choice of pharmacy was affected by the way they were dealt with by pharmacists and pharmacy staff. Much can be learned from those pharmacists with a high number of drug users, who manage to attain good relationships with their clients. Positive handling is a key factor. Drug users like to be treated like "other customers" so that there is no visible evidence to another customer that they are a drug user. In pharmacies with a high number of drug users they may even be treated better than other customers in some ways. Several of these features were identified in the study of drug users (Matheson, 1998b). Since drug users were regular, frequent pharmacy clients there was a level of familiarity which did not exist with other customers/clients. For example drug users and pharmacists often called each other by their first name and there may have been more casual "chat" when a regular drug user collected a prescription compared to other clients.

Privacy in the pharmacy

Stigmatisation was closely related to the level of privacy in the pharmacy. When asked for their views on privacy many drug users were satisfied with the level of privacy in their current pharmacy (Matheson, 1998a). However, for others, privacy, was not an issue because they either did not feel embarrassed themselves or accepted that using public services such as a pharmacy was part of receiving treatment as a drug user.

> *"it just comes wi the territory [of being a drug user]"*

As with stigmatisation, views of privacy were influenced by the visibility of obtaining a prescription. Most of those interviewees who had a "take away" prescription felt there were no visible signs of what their prescriptions were for, so did not feel a lack of privacy was an issue. However, a few of those with 'take away' prescriptions still felt self-conscious. Although this may have been in the mind of the user it may also have been due to a more subtle, visible sign such as having the prescription handed over by the pharmacist as opposed to the staff, which is often the norm with other prescriptions.

> *"The pharmacist can only gi [give] you the methadone. Naebody [nobody] else ken [you know] what I mean? And the pharmacist says 'Here you go' and they [other customers] are sort of saying 'How come he gets the pharmacist giving him that?' ... "*

Users' perceptions of pharmacist motivations

Asking drug users why they thought pharmacists provided services for drug misusers (such as methadone dispensing or needle/syringe exchange services) gave interesting and varied responses. A large proportion believed the decision was out of the pharmacists' hands, that the pharmacists did not have any choice. Of these, some believed that it was the doctor's decision, particularly for methadone dispensing, and that pharmacists simply had to comply with the doctor's wishes. Similarly, others believed it was a government decision and health professionals, whether doctors or pharmacists, had to comply.

> *"because the Government think they can control a drug habit by ... so they say to doctors 'you give it'. I mean somebody's got to somewhere. If the doctors are prescribing it, someone has got to produce it"*

Some believed that pharmacists must be motivated by money and others considered it as a more pragmatic decision simply related to there being a local need for such services. Alternatively several believed that pharmacists had more caring motives such as wanting to help people, wanting to prevent harm, or feeling sorry for drug users as this interview quote illustrated:

> *"I do think that they must sometimes feel quite sorry for people like, their hearts go out to people, watching them ... "*

Views of pharmacists' motivation should be considered in light of their comments on their handling in pharmacies. However, there was no evidence that those who considered pharmacists to be motivated by money as opposed to more altruistic motives had greater experience of negative handling.

THE IDEAL PHARMACY SERVICES
Improvements to pharmacy services

Suggested improvements to pharmacy services were related to drug users' views of what made a good and bad pharmacy service, which in turn was related to their own experiences. As already discussed, drug users often used pharmacies where they felt well-treated. This implied that those pharmacies that are managing a lot of drug users are probably providing a "good" service, according to users. However drug users' expectations affected their views of services. There was evidence that drug users (like other patients/customers) had fairly low expectations of pharmacies which may have been seen as just a place to collect a prescription, or supplies of injecting equipment (Matheson, 1998c). Sheridan and Barber (1996) similarly found that drug users had a low expectation of professional services from pharmacies. This was related to their having rarely been offered advice or information by pharmacists on drug use or safer injecting.

A good pharmacy was often considered as a pharmacy which had friendly, approachable staff (Matheson, 1998c) and a desired improvement to some particular pharmacies was, correspondingly, to improve negative attitudes and overcome the stigmatisation of drug users. A bad pharmacy service was considered as one in which clients were kept waiting unduly perhaps because prescriptions were not made up in advance or because staff may be busy. Therefore, not having to wait for services was greatly appreciated. The need for privacy was important – not necessarily through having a specific private area, but perhaps through discrete handling by the pharmacist. Greater availability of injecting equipment was also considered a potential improvement.

Implications for pharmacy practice

This chapter has explored the drug user's perspective of pharmacy services based on interviews conducted with drug users in research projects. In concluding it is important to consider how pharmacy practice can adapt to take these views into account. There are some general suggestions that individual practitioners can take on board, but also issues that could be addressed at a health care trust or professional level. More detailed practical issues are covered in Chapter 10.

General recommendations for practice, based on research findings, include handling drug users quickly and discreetly to avoid frustration or embarrassment which can then lead to negative responses from the drug users. First visits are often prolonged by having to explain "rules", as part of contracts/agreements; however, if this is handled in a friendly, non-judgmental way, embarrassment and irritation will be minimised. If practitioners do not provide a service which is requested (such as supervised self-administration of methadone), they could give a brief explanation of why not and suggest an alternative pharmacy. Practitioners can give guidance on when is a good or bad time of day to pick up prescriptions, explaining that this would reduce the chance of having to wait for services. However it is important to bear in mind that some drug users, particularly those requiring supervised self-administration, like to take their methadone at a particular time, either first thing in the morning, because they feel they really need it, or as late as possible in the day to help them sleep. If pharmacists get to know individuals, it can allow them to treat that person in a way that will benefit both patient and pharmacist in the long run. A friendly, non-judgmental pharmacist and staff can help an individual rebuild confidence which can be such an important aspect of helping the drug user eventually regain some degree of control of their life.

At a professional or health trust level, there could be (and have been) initiatives to change attitudes by increasing understanding and to develop guidelines to ensure good practice is clarified (see Chapter 5). These initiatives, along with the continuing aggregation of experience in this relatively new aspect of practice, will "normalise" services to drug users and correspondingly reduce the incidence of negative attitudes and the stigmatisation of drug users.

CONCLUSION

This chapter illustrated that the effect of the pharmacist and staff on the drug-using client can be considerable. In many respects drug users are no different from other pharmacy clients, for example, in the way they choose which pharmacy to use, or whether they seek advice on general health issues. However, there are areas in which drug users differ from other clients and that is in their need to be treated discreetly, quickly and, most of all, in a friendly non-judgemental manner. This is because of the stigma attached to being a drug user and the potential conflict of a stigmatised group using what can be a very public amenity – a community pharmacy. Input from an understanding pharmacist can have a considerable effect on whether drug users stay in treatment and eventually take some control of their situation.

ACKNOWLEDGEMENTS

I would like to acknowledge my colleagues Professor Christine Bond, University of Aberdeen Department of General Practice and Primary Care, Professor Neil McKeganey and Dr Joanne Neale from the Centre for Drug Misuse Research, University of Glasgow, for their vital roles in the research project upon which much of this chapter is based.

REFERENCES

Matheson C (1998a). Privacy and stigma in the pharmacy: the illicit drug user's perspective and implications for pharmacy practice. *Pharmaceutical Journal*, 260, 639–641.

Matheson C (1998b). Views of illicit drug users on their treatment and behaviour in Scottish community pharmacies: implication for the harm reduction strategy. *Health Education Journal*, 57, 31–41.

Matheson C (1998c). Illicit drug users, views of a "good" and "bad" pharmacy service. *Journal of Social and Administrative Pharmacy*, 15, 104–112.

Matheson C, Bond CM, Hickey F (1999). Prescribing and dispensing for drug misusers in primary care: current practice in Scotland. *Family Practice*, 16, 375–379.

Matheson C, Bond C, Paitcairn J (In press). Community pharmacy services for drug misusers: what difference does five years make? *Addiction*.

Neale J (1998a). Reducing Risks: drug users, views of accessing and disposing of injecting equipment. *Addiction Research*, 6, 147–163.

Neale J (1998b). Drug users' views of prescribed methadone. *Drugs: Education, Prevention and Policy*, 5, 33–45.

Neale J (1999). Drug Users' Views of substitute prescribing conditions. *International Journal of Drug Policy*, 10, 247–258.

Royal Pharmaceutical Society (1997). *Royal Pharmaceutical Society Standards and Practice Advice Notes*, RPSGB, London.

Sheridan J, Barber N (1996). Drug misusers' experiences and opinions of community pharmacists and community pharmacy services. *Pharmaceutical Journal*, 257, 325–327.

Sheridan J, Lovell S, Turnbull P, Parsons J, Stimson G, Strang J (2000). Pharmacy-based needle exchange (PBNX) scheme in South-East England: Survey of service providers. *Addiction*, 95, 1551–1560.

Strang J, Sheridan J, Barber N (1996). Prescribing injectable and oral methadone to opiate addicts: results from the 1995 national postal survey of community pharmacies in England and Wales. *British Medical Journal*, 313, 270–272.

9

Legal and ethical considerations for community pharmacists in the United Kingdom

Kay Roberts

INTRODUCTION

Community pharmacists are uniquely placed to provide services to drug users. Furthermore, as specialists in the composition and use of medicines, they are able to provide accurate, up to date, and appropriate information to clients and health care professionals. They are able to supply medicines prescribed for the treatment of substance dependence and, if necessary, ancillary equipment such as syringes, needles and health promotion literature. Community pharmacists are accessible to the public, without appointment – typically for about nine hours a day, five, six or seven days a week.

However, they are subject to legal and ethical restrictions that can affect the extent to which they are able to provide such services. As demonstrated in Chapter 3, the degree to which pharmacists (and community pharmacists in particular) have been involved in services to drug misusers has been, to a large extent, determined by changes in drugs legislation as well as by changes in the manner in which health care in the United Kingdom is provided and funded. The legal and ethical restrictions to which pharmacists are subjected can, on occasion, cause frustration and lack of understanding on the part of clients, prescribing doctors and other workers in the field of substance misuse.

This chapter will consider the practical implications for community pharmacists and others arising from United Kingdom and international legislation controlling the availability and supply of drugs, and the UK pharmacists' Code of Ethics. The impact of both of these on the practice of pharmacy and the optimum provision of pharmaceutical services to drug users will also be discussed. Issues that will be addressed include the supply and administration of drugs used in the treatment of drug dependence, pharmacists' involvement in needle and syringe exchange schemes, confidentiality, privacy in the pharmacy, pharmacists as members of the public, and services to under 16 year olds. Although most of the consideration of legislation and ethics focuses on practice in the United Kingdom, parallels can, in most cases, be drawn to experience elsewhere.

LEGISLATION IN GREAT BRITAIN

As mentioned in Chapter 3, since the nineteenth century there have been many national and international attempts to control the use of certain drugs and to prevent their misuse by the public. For pharmacists in the United Kingdom, the main Acts and Regulations that currently govern their ability to supply and sell medicines which contain drugs liable to misuse are: the Misuse of Drugs Act 1971, the Misuse of Drugs Regulations 1985 and amendments, the Drug Trafficking Offences Act 1986 and the Medicines Act 1968 and its Regulations. It is often when two or more of these Acts and Regulations apply that problems and misunderstandings can occur.

The Misuse of Drugs Act 1971 controls the supply, prescription and administration of "dangerous and other harmful drugs" which are designated as "Controlled Drugs"(CDs). The aim of this Act is to prevent the misuse of CDs by imposing restrictions on their possession, supply, manufacture, import or export except as allowed for by regulations or licence from the Secretary of State. The use of CDs as medicines is permitted by the Misuse of Drugs Regulations 1985, as amended. Other Misuse of Drugs Regulations that impact on pharmacy are those covering the safe custody of CDs and the requirements for the writing of prescriptions. Over the past twenty or so years, the scope of the Misuse of Drugs Act 1971 and its regulations have been amended to reflect international legislation and conventions and the specific drugs which are currently causing concern. The Act now covers many psychotropic drugs not available or not known to be misused at the time the Act was first formulated.

By virtue of Section 34 of the Drug Trafficking Offences Act 1986, Section 9A of the Misuse of Drugs Act makes it an offence for anyone to knowingly sell or supply products that can be used for the preparation or administration of a Controlled substance. In theory, this means that the sale or supply of swabs, filters, water for injection, citric or ascorbic acid to someone a pharmacist knows or suspects will use them for such a purpose would be a contravention of the Act. Needles and syringes are specifically exempted from Section 9A.

The Misuse of Drugs Regulations 1985 classify substances into five schedules according to different levels of control. Schedule 1 includes hallucinogenic drugs such as LSD and cannabis that are considered to have virtually no recognised therapeutic use. Production and supply of drugs in this schedule are limited to purposes of research or other special purposes. At the time of going to press, there is much discussion in the United Kingdom surrounding the use of cannabis for medical purposes, in particular, whether or not the drug has a role in the treatment of multiple sclerosis, glaucoma and chemotherapy-induced nausea (Strang *et al.*, 2000a).

Schedules 2 to 5 relate to drugs or substances used in treatment. Therefore, community pharmacists need to be fully cognisant of the details of the regulations pertaining to them, as these determine whether or not a drug may be sold or supplied on the prescription of a doctor or dentist, what records are required to be kept, whether safe storage is required, (i.e. in the CD cabinet) and whether or not licences are required for import and export. A comprehensive summary of the legal requirements for CDs as they apply to pharmacists can be found in the Royal Pharmaceutical Society of Great Britain's (RPSGB) publication: *Medicines, Ethics and Practice: A Guide for Pharmacists* (MEPG) (RPSGB, 2002) that is updated every six months and routinely sent to all pharmacists. Fact sheets on "Controlled Drugs in Community Pharmacy" and the "Export of Medicines" are available from the RPSGB Law Department.

The Medicines Act 1968 and its Regulations control the sale, supply and administration of both prescription and over-the-counter "OTC" medicines. Medicines are designated as Prescription Only Medicine [POM], Pharmacy Medicine [P] or General Sale List [GSL]. Medicines whose ingredients are covered by Schedules 2 to 4 of the Misuse of Drugs Regulations are designated as POMs. Schedule 5 of the Misuse of Drugs Regulations contains preparations of certain CDs, for example codeine, pholcodine, morphine that are exempt from full control when present in medicinal products of low strength. There is currently no United Kingdom restriction on the import, export, possession or administration of Schedule 5 preparations (into the UK) and safe custody requirements do not apply. However, this does not mean that the same exemptions apply in other countries. Community pharmacists need to be aware of this when, for instance, they sell or supply products containing codeine to persons going abroad either for work or holiday. Some countries, even within the European Union, do not allow the importation of products containing codeine.

THE PHARMACISTS' PROFESSIONAL CODE OF ETHICS

Pharmacists practising their profession in Great Britain are required to adhere to the Code of Ethics and Professional Standards laid down by the RPSGB. Other national Pharmaceutical Societies expect similar professional standards to be maintained by their members. However, it needs to be recognised that the RPSGB "is unique in the world of pharmacy bodies in having not two, but three separate roles – professional, regulatory and law enforcement" (Ferguson, 2000). In order to practise, pharmacists in Britain must register annually with the RPSGB. The RPSGB, through its Statutory Committee, has the power to strike a pharmacist off its register and thus disqualify him or her from practice. Over the years, many of the offences that bring pharmacists in front of the Statutory Committee related to the provisions of the Misuse of Drugs Act and its Regulations. Compliance with the Society's Code of Professional Ethics may also be taken into consideration when the outcome of a particular case is determined.

The Code of Ethics consists of two parts with nine principles that are supplemented by more detailed obligations. Together these set out the fundamental duties that apply to all British pharmacists. The Code of Ethics is supported by Guidance that is published in the form of the MEPG. It is intended to help in the interpretation of the Code, is published every six months to include amendments and is sent to all registered pharmacists as a matter of course. However, it is recognised that guidance cannot cover every situation. When in doubt, pharmacists are urged to seek further advice from the Society's Professional Standards Directorate.

As well as comprehensively covering the various requirements of the Misuse of Drugs Legislation, the MEPG includes practical advice and raises pharmacists' awareness of a range of products that are available from pharmacies and which could be misused. The advice warns that pharmacists should be aware of any problems in their area, whether or not they are general, and that almost any substance can be misused and that the list provided in the guidance is not exhaustive.

The rest of this chapter will look at some of the professional and ethical dilemmas which community pharmacists face.

GUIDELINES FOR THE CARE AND TREATMENT OF DRUG MISUSERS

Pharmacists and other health professionals involved in the provision of services to drug misusers should be aware of any national or local guidance. In the United Kingdom, the Departments of Health published comprehensive guidance on the clinical management of drug misusers (Departments of Health, 1999). This document is not only full of practical guidance, but it is also a very useful reference source. In addition to this, the four UK Departments of Health issue guidance from time to time on the provision of services. This advice is then implemented at local level by the local health authorities. Local pharmaceutical committees may issue guidance to cover the pharmaceutical issues relating to a supervised methadone programme or needle and syringe exchange scheme in their area. Pharmacists should also be aware of any local guidance that has been issued to medical colleagues. It is helpful to ensure that matters of shared interest, such as the writing of prescriptions, are common to both sets of advice.

Other specific advice for pharmacists around pharmaceutical services for drug misusers is contained in MEPG.

CONFIDENTIALITY AND PRIVACY

The Code of Ethics is specific about confidentiality for all patients and this obviously includes drug misusers. Confidentiality issues are threefold: the first issue relates to sharing of information between other professionals (see later), the second relates to the privacy afforded an individual when they are discussing sensitive matters, such as the use of illicit drugs, and the third relates to discussing patients/clients outside the work environment. Drug workers and others caring for those who use drugs are often critical of the poor level of privacy and confidentiality that their clients receive in pharmacies. Pharmacists and their staff need to remember that methadone patients have the same rights as other users of the pharmacy. Every customer should be treated with courtesy and respect. There are no grounds for treating patients on a methadone programme as "second-class citizens".

Confidentiality

The ability of pharmacists to maintain patient confidentiality is a source of some concern to workers in the field of substance misuse as well as drug users themselves. Drug workers and drug users are often unaware that the pharmacists' Code of Ethics requires them to respect the confidentiality of information acquired in the course of professional practice that relates to a patient and the patient's family. The need to ensure patient confidentiality is very important to most drug users. Family, friends and neighbours may be unaware of the situation and the patient will not wish to be further stigmatised.

However, there will be occasions when, in the best interests of the patient, information will need to be shared between health professionals and drug workers. Whenever possible, this should have been done with the patients' knowledge and permission.

Exceptions to this rule would be when a coroner, judge or other presiding officer of a court directs disclosure of information. Confidential information should not be disclosed to a policeman, social worker, solicitor or court official except as directed by the presiding officer or with the consent of the patient concerned. Other exceptions would be to prevent serious injury or risk to public health, or to assist the prevention, detection or prosecution of a serious crime. In the case of exceptions the pharmacist will need to assess the risk of disclosure against the rights of the patient to confidentiality, and would be wise to seek advice (if possible) and to document, at the time, the basis for their decision.

Sharing of information

Situations may well arise when it is appropriate and necessary to share information about a patient with the prescribing doctor or drug worker. Any written or verbal agreement or contract which the pharmacist has with the patient should make it absolutely clear that these situations may occur and what action will be taken. For instance, in the interests of the patient's safety, it will be necessary to discuss missed doses, intoxication, deterioration of health with the prescribing doctor, as an alteration in dose may be necessary. Some "patient contracts/agreements" between prescribing doctor and patient include "good behaviour" in the pharmacy as a condition for continued treatment. When reporting problematic behaviour, the pharmacist will need to consider each incident on its merits and decide whether or not it is appropriate to take the matter further.

Privacy

In recent years there has been an increasing awareness of the need provide a quiet area where questions can be asked and advice given without the conversation being overheard. The need for such an area is particularly relevant to the supervised administration of methadone and other medicines and the supply of clean injecting equipment as part of a needle and syringe exchange scheme. The area provided should be used as an advice/consultation area for all customers. It is also important that the area is not so enclosed that customers are deterred from using it.

INSTALMENT DISPENSING AND MISSED DOSES OF METHADONE

In many countries other than the UK that have methadone programmes, clients receive their medication in daily instalments, and consume it on the pharmacy premises under the supervision of a pharmacist. "Take-home" doses are normally only available at weekends and over public holiday periods. The aim of such frequent supervised instalment dispensing is to prevent or reduce leakage of methadone onto the illegal market and to prevent inadvertent overdose by non-tolerant individuals. However, doctors in the UK can and do prescribe for any period of time (e.g. daily, weekly, twice a week). "Take-home" doses are the norm for most patients and UK pharmacists can be faced with difficult legal and ethical situations as a result of such dispensing requirements, due to the stringent nature of the Misuse of Drugs Regulations.

Legal issues

All prescriptions for CDs in the UK must conform to Regulations 15 and 16 of the Misuse of Drugs Regulations. In brief, this means that prescriptions must be written according to set rules and that prescriptions which do not conform to such rules are not legal and must not be dispensed until amended by the prescribing doctor. In addition, the number of instalments per week, on which days and the daily dose must be specified. Pharmacists are not allowed to deviate from these instructions – for example by substituting sugar-free formulations for the normal formulation, or dispensing instalments in advance of the date specified. The strictness of these regulations often brings pharmacists into conflict with drug users who may wish to have doses dispensed in advance of the doctor's instructions, or to obtain doses which they failed to collect, neither of these options allowed under the regulations.

Often instructions are unclear or even omitted. A recent court case in England confirmed the fact that responsibility for the legality and clarity of a prescription falls squarely on the supplier of the medicines and not the prescribing doctor (Gordon Appelbe, 1999). This means that pharmacists should contact the prescribing doctor in order to clarify instructions. In practice, patients and prescribing doctors are often irritated by what they perceive as unnecessary strict adherence to the law on the part of the pharmacist.

Duty of care

Pharmacists owe a duty of care to their customers. A duty of care arises when the pharmacist can reasonably foresee that the patient is likely to suffer harm from his/her conduct. The MEPG states that, within a pharmacy, the pharmacist owes a duty of care to anyone s/he can reasonably foresee is likely to suffer harm from his/her conduct e.g. liability for professional services such as dispensing, deficient advice, liability for the safety of customers coming onto the pharmacy premises (occupiers' liability). In the case of instalment dispensing this would relate to situations where a patient is intoxicated or has missed several doses of methadone and may have an attenuated tolerance to opiates, thus putting them at an increased risk of overdose.

Problem which can arise

A methadone client in a state of withdrawal because of a missed dose can become irate and difficult. Trying to explain to such a person that a "missed dose of methadone" cannot be supplied may often prove difficult and, sometimes, even dangerous. On occasions pharmacists and their staff have been threatened or subjected to abuse. Even where the patient has been previously advised that missed doses cannot be dispensed retrospectively, they can become angry and abusive when confronted by a pharmacist who is legally unable to provide the missed dose. It is important for pharmacists to ensure that they and their staff are aware of the possibility of such situations and be able to deal with them in an appropriate manner (see Chapter 11).

Other matters that need to be taken into account in relation to missed doses of methadone:

- dose missed because patient failed to present prescription on time. If starting date is stated on prescription then first dose is due on that date. If the patient does not present the prescription until one or two days later, for instance, then the missed doses cannot be dispensed.
- doses (especially weekend) not collected because patient in police custody. The missed doses will be forfeit. Some local police forces allow collection of doses from the pharmacy by an agent (usually a police officer). Such procedures prevent

doses being missed and tolerance being lost (see below for collection of CDs by a representative).

SUPERVISION OF CONSUMPTION OF CDs
IN THE PHARMACY
Legal issues

There is currently no legal requirement under the UK Misuse of Drugs or the Medicines Acts for doses of methadone to be supervised or even prescribed by daily instalment (Departments of Health, 1999). In other words, supervised consumption of methadone or any other medication for patients attending a pharmacy has no basis in British law. It is a voluntary undertaking on behalf of the pharmacist and client. However, prescribing doctors would be understandably annoyed if supervision did not take place if they had specifically requested it on a prescription. In addition, fellow pharmacists become irritated if they see that attempts to prevent the leakage of methadone onto the streets are undermined by those colleagues who choose to ignore the prescribing doctors' instructions.

In some areas, local schemes have been set up to provide this service (e.g. Gruer *et al.*, 1997). If the pharmacist is not part of a local scheme, then the options are either to supervise consumption for the patient or advise him/her to take the prescription to a colleague who does supervise. Hopefully, where a scheme does exist, such an eventuality as described would not arise because the prescribing doctor will have contacted the pharmacist in advance of the patient presenting the prescription to ensure that supervision is possible.

It is normally understood that pharmacists will abide by the prescribing doctor's instructions. In addition, those pharmacists who have a contract with their local health authority to undertake supervision could be in breach of contract if they did not undertake the service specified in the contract. However, there are occasions when it would be inappropriate either to supply or supervise consumption of methadone:

- when the patient presents in the pharmacy in an intoxicated state;
- when the patient has not collected his or her prescribed dose for three or more consecutive days and may have depleted tolerance to opiates.

Ethical issues

One potential issue that could lead to a breach of duty of care arises when a pharmacist supervises the consumption of methadone in the pharmacy, when the client is in an "unfit" state. Pharmacists should ensure that the patient is in a fit state to take the dose. There is a potential for overdose if a dose of methadone is administered to an intoxicated patient or to a patient who has missed several doses and has (through temporary abstinence of days or weeks) lost tolerance to opiates.

Pharmacists supervising consumption of any medication on their premises need to be aware that they could be held to be responsible if the patient suffers harm as a result of their actions. The general standard of care is taken to be that of a "prudent and reasonable man". However, where the person has undertaken an activity that requires special skill, s/he will be expected to show the level of skill one would expect from a reasonably competent person undertaking activities of a similar nature.

It would be difficult to argue in court that a fatal dose of methadone was administered to an intoxicated or intolerant individual "because the prescription required it".

Additional difficulties

As mentioned above, prescriptions for a CD must contain clear instructions around instalments, and prescribing doctors should inform pharmacists if they wish the prescription to be dispensed under supervision. Ideally, the prescribing doctor should ascertain from the patient which pharmacy they wish to attend, and then the pharmacist should be contacted to ensure that they are able and willing to supervise consumption. In the event of a prescription requesting supervision being received by a "non-supervising" pharmacy, the prescribing doctor should be contacted and the situation explained. It is inadvisable for the patient to be allowed to "take away" the prescribed dose where supervision has been requested. If necessary, the patient could be advised of the nearest pharmacy that does carry out supervision.

Other difficulties may arise, for example, when a regular patient claiming sickness says they would be grateful if the dose was not supervised that day. "Can you allow a 'take-away dose' just this once?" Although there is no requirement in law for a methadone prescription to specify whether or not the dose should be subject to supervised consumption, it would not be good practice to ignore the prescribing doctor's instructions. If the patient or any one else suffered harm as a result of allowing "take-home doses" in this circumstance, it would be difficult for the pharmacist to defend his/her actions. In addition, it is important to remember that one aim of a supervised methadone service is to reduce "leakage" or "spillage" of drugs liable to misuse into the community. In these circumstances, the pharmacist may be wiser to speak on the telephone to the prescribing doctor (or the drug team) to ascertain their advice with regard to the patient's request.

TRAVELLING ABROAD WITH CDs:
"Over-the-counter medicines" which contain Schedule 5 CDs – legal issues

There are no UK restrictions on the import or export of medicines contained in Schedule 5 of the Misuse of Drugs Regulations. Products included in this category contain small quantities of substances such as codeine, pholcodine, dihydrocodeine or morphine. However, it must be remembered that the legislation in other countries may not be identical. It is advisable for pharmacists to alert travellers to the fact, even though they are allowed to take these products out of the UK, it may be illegal in the law of the other country to which they are travelling to import products containing such ingredients.

Ethical issues

It would be helpful if pharmacists gave advice to their customers on travelling abroad with medicines, whether purchased or prescribed. They could save them inconvenience and embarrassment if they supplied practical advice in advance of travel. Another ethical issue for pharmacists to consider is "trafficking" in medicines that have the potential for misuse. Pharmacists should be alert to the potential for sale abroad by customers purchasing unusually large quantities of OTC medicines containing codeine, or ephedrine prior to travelling abroad. Further issues relating to the overuse or misuse of OTC medications are considered in Chapter 13.

Patients on methadone and other prescribed CDs wishing to travel abroad – legal issues

Patients intending to carry Schedule 2 (e.g. methadone) or schedule 3 (e.g. temazepam) drugs abroad may require an export licence. Such a licence is dependent on the amount of drug to be imported or exported. Further details are available from the Home Office. Licences, once granted, do not have any legal status outside the UK and are only issued to facilitate passage through UK Customs control. For clearance in the country to be visited it is necessary to approach that country's embassy or High Commission in the UK.

Both the prescribing doctor and the pharmacist could be asked for advice by methadone patients wishing to go abroad. It needs to be recognised that such patients have the same rights to holidays as other people. Patients should be given the necessary advice and reminded that they will need to allow plenty of time for the appropriate licences to be granted by the Home Office or the authorities in the country to which they are travelling. A letter from the prescribing doctor will be insufficient. Both patient and prescribing doctor need to be aware that only a limited amount of methadone can be exported. This fact may well limit the time that the patient can spend abroad if it is not possible to arrange for continuation of the treatment in the country of destination. Because of the inconvenience of travelling with methadone mixture, the patient might request a change to tablets or even ampoules. There is a need to be aware of the resale value of such formulations onto the illicit market and the fact that tablets may be crushed and injected (which can cause major problems at injecting sites), before a decision is made to alter the formulation.

PATIENT IDENTITY

In 1997 a pharmacist was referred to the Statutory Committee for allegedly supplying a prescription to the wrong patient and failing to take remedial action (Law and Ethics Bulletin, 1997). A recent incident in Glasgow has highlighted the need for pharmacists to ensure that the person presenting a prescription for methadone (whether supervised or not) is the person to whom the prescription belongs. In the incident in question, a new patient presented a prescription for supervised methadone. The pharmacist contacted the doctor to confirm the authenticity of the prescription, which was dispensed according to the prescribing doctor's instructions. Unfortunately, unbeknown to the pharmacist, the original patient had sold his prescription to someone else who then presented the prescription at the pharmacy. The prescription was genuine, but the patient was not. It may be that some form of identification should be available so that patients' identity can be checked when they first present at a pharmacy.

The practice advice section of the MEP guide suggests that pharmacists should consider a method of patient identification (e.g. record card for each patient). However, whether such an initiative is generally considered to be acceptable to the patient (from the point of view of civil liberties) seems to vary from one area to another. Perhaps it could be put to the patient that it is in their interest to ensure that others do not abuse their dose.

As mentioned previously in this chapter, the pharmacist has a duty of care to the patient and therefore must take sufficient steps to ensure that prescriptions are not inadvertently supplied to the wrong patient. This could have particular implications where the patient is consuming the methadone under the supervision of the pharmacist.

SUBSTITUTION OF COLOURLESS AND/OR SUGAR-FREE METHADONE MIXTURE ON PRESCRIPTIONS
Legal issues
In the UK, the introduction of different presentations of methadone mixture, such as colourless or sugar-free, has resulted in patients requesting pharmacists to substitute one formulation for the other. A recent RPSGB Law and Ethics bulletin reminded pharmacists of the importance of dispensing exactly what the prescription specifies (Law and Ethics Bulletin, 1999). The Bulletin advises that sugar-free or colourless presentations may only be dispensed if so specified on the prescription and that the prescribing doctor must make any alterations. It is worth bearing in mind that there is anecdotal evidence to suggest that it is easier to inject sugar-free methadone solutions than it is to inject the standard sugar-based formulation.

Many drug users blame methadone syrup for the state of their teeth. However, it is more likely that the combined effects of opiates, poor oral hygiene and poor nutrition have taken their toll. Advice to patients on how to avoid further decay should be made available, including rinsing the mouth out with water after drinking the methadone, using sugar-free gum, good oral hygiene practices and getting regular check-ups with the dentist. Further aspects of dental health are dealt with in Chapter 13.

CHILD SAFETY – SAFE STORAGE OF MEDICINES
Legal issues
As mentioned above, pharmacists have a duty of care to their customers and patients. They should ensure that appropriate warnings and advice are given to patients, parents and carers to ensure that medications supplied by them do not cause accidental poisoning of children. This is particularly a cause for concern since each daily dose for the patient is potentially a lethal dose for an opiate-intolerant child. Furthermore, opiate dependent patients often use severely insufficient precautions about storage of take-home doses of methadone at home (Calman *et al.*, 1996).

Ethical issues
The RPSGB Standards of Good Professional Practice requires that all solid dose and all oral and external liquid preparations must be dispensed in a reclosable child resistant container (CRC), unless the medicine is in an original pack. Other exceptions include patients who have problems opening CRCs or if no suitable CRC is available for a particular liquid formulation. In such cases additional advice must be given to ensure that all medicines are kept out of the reach of children. The majority of methadone prescribed in the UK is in a liquid formulation and all dispensed bottles will need to have a CRC.

Preventing risk of child overdose
There have been several unfortunate instances where children have died as a result of ingesting methadone mixture intended for a parent (Binchy *et al.*, 1994). Every effort should be made to ensure that "take-away" doses of methadone do not get into

the hands of children. Warning labels and specially designed stickers on the dispensing container, leaflets and extra advice at the point of dispensing should be provided. Such initiatives are particularly important when large volumes of methadone are being given out e.g. at times of public and other holiday periods.

Care must also be taken to ensure that CRCs are used properly. Problems can arise if the tops are not locked closed, if the bottle neck and cap are not kept clean and free from sugar granules, or the patient or carer transfers the medication from the CRC to another non-CRC container for easier access. The correct type of CRC needs to be used for liquid medications to prevent leakage from the cap.

When a large number of doses are dispensed in one bottle, the pharmacist should ensure the patient has a suitable means of measuring out each day's dose. Research in Ireland showed that a number of clients used babies' bottles to measure out methadone, with the obvious potential for accidental overdoses to occur in babies fed from uncleaned bottles (Harkin *et al.*, 1999).

COLLECTION OF CDs BY PATIENT'S REPRESENTATIVE
Legal issues
The Misuse of Drugs Regulations allow the possession of a CD by a person who is conveying it to another person who is authorised to possess the drug. Thus it is legal for a representative (agent) to collect a CD prescription on behalf of the patient for whom it was prescribed. However, a letter of authority from the patient is required.

Ethical issues
When the prescription being collected is for the treatment of drug dependence there is the possibility that the medicine may not reach the person for whom it was intended, as such drugs have a "black market" value. The RPSGB Law Department has suggested that pharmacists request a "letter of authority" from the patient before making a supply to his/her agent (Law and Ethics Bulletin, 1996). Pharmacists are advised of the need to ensure that the letters of authority are genuine and should be wary of patients that use different agents. A separate "letter of authority" from the patient should be obtained on each occasion a supply is made to an agent. Letters should be retained for a period of time so that a comparison of signatures can be undertaken. It is also good practice to have arrangements with local prescribing doctors about collection of methadone by agents.

Practical issues
There may well be genuine reasons why a drug-using patient is unable to attend the pharmacy in person, as, for example, when in police custody or when too ill to leave home. It is in the pharmacist's interest to ensure that supplies in such circumstances are genuine and documented.

In the case of supplies to an agent where the prescribing doctor has requested supervised consumption in the pharmacy, the patient needs to be aware that it is probably essential, and certainly wise, for the pharmacist to speak to the doctor before supply to an agent can be made, as an alteration to the prescribing doctor's instructions has been requested. It would be advantageous to both pharmacists and prescribing doctors to include a clause to this effect in any written or verbal agreement with the patient.

One occasion when an unsupervised supply to an agent may be necessary is when the patient is being held in police custody. A pharmacist may supply doses of methadone to a police officer acting as agent for the patient. However, the pharmacist may only supply the methadone in accordance with the prescribing doctor's directions about the amount of instalment to be dispensed and the intervals to be observed when supplying. In these circumstances the police officer is acting as the patient's representative (agent) and is authorised by Regulations 6(2) and 7(f) of the Misuse of Drugs Regulations to convey the medicine to the patient. However, the Police and Criminal Evidence Act 1984 Code of Practice states that no police officer may administer [to a detained person] medicines that are CDs. These can only be administered by a police surgeon or, if the police surgeon so advises, be self-administered by the detainee. In the latter case, the custody officer could be said to be supervising the consumption of the dose.

PROVISION OF SERVICES TO THOSE UNDER 16 YEARS OF AGE

Pharmacists and others involved in the treatment of drug misuse are understandably concerned when dealing with young people under the age of sixteen years. In its 1998 report, the RPSGB Working Party on Pharmaceutical Services for Drug Misusers recommended that community pharmacists needed guidelines on the provision of needle and syringe exchange services and advice on sexual health to those under the age of sixteen years (RPSGB, 1998). Both the Standing Conference on Drug Abuse (Dale-Perera *et al.*, 1999) and the Scottish Drugs Forum (1999) have published policy guidance for those working with young drug users. As there are important differences between English and Scottish Law that are relevant to this issue, it is important to refer to the version most appropriate for your practice.

Legal issues

Both sets of guidance stress that in accordance with the Children Act 1989, the Children (Scotland) Act 1995 and the UN Convention on the Child (1989), the welfare of the child is of paramount importance. An additional piece of legislation for Scottish practitioners is the Age of Legal Capacity (Scotland) Act 1991. The framework of the Scottish Legislation respects the privacy and dignity of young people, their right to make certain decisions for themselves and the right to a say in who should and should not be involved in their care.

Ethical issues

Principle four of the RPSGB Code of Ethics states that a pharmacist must respect the confidentiality of information acquired in the course of professional practice relating to a patient or a patient's family. It goes on to say that such information must not be disclosed to anyone without the consent of the patient or appropriate guardian unless there is a major interest of the patient or the public that requires such disclosure. The guidance to this principle states that where the patient is a child, the pharmacist may have to decide whether to release information to a parent or guardian without the consent of the child, if such disclosure would be in the best interests of the child. Such a decision will depend on the maturity of the child concerned and his/her relationship with parent or guardian. When deciding on the best way forward, pharmacists should bear in mind the legal rights of the child concerned.

If in doubt, pharmacists may find it helpful to contact local needle exchange co-ordinators, local pharmaceutical advisors or the local drugs team for advice. Further advice can be sought from the RPSGB Professional Standards Directorate. Final decision, however, rests with the professional judgement of pharmacist after all the circumstances have been taken into account.

Appendix six of the 1999 Departments of Health guidelines on clinical treatment gives comprehensive advice on issues surrounding the treatment of young people with drug misuse problems. The guidance states that only in exceptional circumstances should GPs prescribe substitute medication to under-16s and then this would be expected to be with the involvement of specialist agencies. The guidance also recognises that in an emergency there may be insufficient time to obtain parental consent to treatment (Departments of Health *et al*, 1999). As far as the dispensing of prescriptions of methadone for those under 16 is concerned, pharmacists are in the same position as they are when they dispense any medicine for a child or young person. It is the prescribing doctor who could be required to justify his/her actions if treatment is undertaken without the knowledge of the parents. In England, the judgement of the House of Lords in the Gillick case (Gillick v West Norfolk and Wisbech Health Authority, 1985) in 1985 provided that doctors may give medical treatment to a child or young person under 16 without parental consent if the doctor finds the particular young person competent ("Gillick competent"). The ability to provide treatment to under-16s has been extended by analogy to certain other professionals. In Scotland, decisions relating to treatment appear to be governed by the Age of Legal Capacity (Scotland) Act 1991. Parental consent is irrelevant unless the child is deemed incapable of understanding. The Gillick judgement is not relevant under Scottish Law.

Pharmacists involved in the provision of services to young people under the age of sixteen need to be aware of the rights of children as well as the rights of the parents. In particular, the right of the child to confidentiality should be maintained. Prescriptions for substitute medication should be treated in the same way as those for other patients. Pharmacists involved in needle exchange schemes should consider the professional, ethical, legal and public health issues carefully before supplying or refusing to supply injecting equipment.

REQUEST FOR INJECTING PARAPHERNALIA BY A KNOWN OR SUSPECTED INJECTING DRUG USER

What are the legal issues?

Under the Drug Trafficking Offences / Misuse of Drugs Acts, "a person who supplies or offers to supply any article which may be used or adapted to be used (whether by itself or in combination with another article or other articles) in the administration by any person of a CD to himself or another believing that the article (or article as adapted) is to be used in circumstances where the administration is unlawful, is guilty of an offence". For most community pharmacists, this is relevant with regard to requests for citric and ascorbic acids, which are used by drug users in the UK and elsewhere in Europe to acidify "brown" heroin ("black market" heroin, typically from South-West Asia) to make it sufficiently soluble for injection (Strang *et al.*, 2000b). The problem for pharmacists is that they may be aware of the intended purpose for which the acids will be used and it is this knowledge that makes the sale of acidifiers an offence under the Misuse of Drugs Act.

Ethical issues

The RPSGB MEPG section on Substances of Misuse reminds pharmacists to be aware that "a pharmacist must exercise professional judgement to prevent the supply of unnecessary or excessive quantities of medicines and other products, particularly those that are liable to misuse...". The section specifically mentions that citric and ascorbic acids are used to convert insoluble street heroin into a form that is more suitable for intravenous injection.

It has been argued that this section of the law was never meant to prevent harm reduction measures, such as the supply of filters, swabs or acidifiers. In England, both the police and the Crown Prosecution Services appear to ignore technical breaches of the legislation. A report in the drug-field magazine *Druglink* (Preston, 1999) describes how the local drug service has secured reassurance from the police and the Crown Prosecution Service that neither investigation nor prosecution was being considered. In response, the RPSGB Law Department has confirmed that, in the absence of a prosecution (or the wider charge of misconduct), it would not discipline members who are in breach of section 9A of the Misuse of Drugs Act. However, it must be recognised that the police and Crown Prosecution Service in other parts of the country could take a different view. Pharmacists are probably best advised to initiate these relevant local discussions and to seek the opinion of their local RPSGB Inspector prior to making citric acid readily available to needle and syringe exchange clients.

A recent decision in Glasgow and Strathkelvin has stated that pharmacists supplying citric acid as part of a needle exchange scheme, will not be prosecuted. This advice has been supported by the Greater Glasgow Drug Action Team, Strathclyde police and the Council of the Royal Pharmaceutical Society. Local pharmacists have now received training in the use of acidifiers as part of a harm reduction programme.

Harm reduction issues

Both citric and ascorbic acids if used in excess can cause local "burning" at the injection site – "citric burns". It is, therefore, essential those drug injectors who use acidifiers know how much to use and how to prepare the products so that the incidence of "citric burns" is minimised. It is important to ensure that, if providing citric or ascorbic acids, advice is given on how much acid to use. The ability of pharmacists and drug workers to offer sound advice on how to minimise "acid burns" could prevent or reduce the incidence of such injuries. It is interesting to note that pharmacists in France have developed small sachets of citric acid that are distributed together with needles, syringes, swabs and vials of sterile water and a small metal "Stericup" that can be used as a "cooker".

CONCLUSION

The ethical and legal dilemmas for community pharmacists are varied and many and this chapter is in no way exhaustive in its coverage of the issues. Furthermore, some of the issues detailed above are specific to the UK context. However, in most cases where such dilemmas appear in practice, a sound knowledge of the law, a contextual understanding of the code of ethics and a firm grasp of the need to exercise a duty of care while remaining within the law are all key to providing a safe, effective, legal and ethical service. Last, but by no means least, is the importance of remembering that drug users are part of the "local community" and deserve to be treated with the same level of respect and professionalism that would be afforded any other member of the community.

REFERENCES

Age of Legal Capacity (Scotland) Act (1991). HMSO, Edinburgh.

Appelbe G (1999). When is an instalment prescription not an instalment prescription. *PharMAGazine*, 2, 5, 2–3.

Binchy JM, Molyneux EM, Manning J (1994). Accidental ingestion of methadone by children in Merseyside. *British Medical Journal*, 308, 1335–1336.

Calman L, Finch E, Powis B, Strang J (1996). Methadone treatment. Only half of patients store methadone in safe place. *British Medical Journal*, 313, 1481.

Children (Scotland) Act (1995). HMSO, Edinburgh.

Children Act (1989). HMSO, London.

Dale-Perera A, Hamilton C, Evans C, Britton J (1999). *Young people and drugs: policy guidance for drug interventions*. Standing Conference on Drug Abuse, London.

Departments of Health *et al.* (1999). *Drug Misuse and Dependence: Guidelines on Clinical Management*, The Stationery Office, London.

Drug Trafficking Offences Act (1986). Section 34. HMSO, London.

Ferguson J (2000). The Pharmaceutical Society – in defence of a unique body. *Pharmaceutical Journal*, 265, 293.

Gillick v West Norfolk and Wisbech Health Authority (1985). 3 All ER 402.

Gruer L, Wilson P, Scott R, Elliott L, Macleod J, Harden K, Forrester E, Hinshelwood S, McNulty H, Silk P (1997). General practitioner centred scheme for treatment of opiate dependent drug injectors in Glasgow. *British Medical Journal*, 314, 1730–1735.

Harkin K, Quinn C, Bradley F (1999). Storing methadone in babies' bottles puts young children at risk (letter). *British Medical Journal*, 318, 329.

Law and Ethics Bulletin (1996). Collection of CDs by agent. *Pharmaceutical Journal*, 256, 677.

Law and Ethics Bulletin (1997). Supply to wrong patient. *Pharmaceutical Journal*, 259, 599.

Law and Ethics Bulletin (1999). Substitution of colourless and/or sugar-free methadone mixture on prescriptions. *Pharmaceutical Journal*, 263, 308.

Medicines Act (1968). HMSO, London.

Misuse of Drugs Act (1971). HMSO, London.

Misuse of Drugs Act 1971 (Modification) Order (1986), Section 9A(1) and Schedule 4. HMSO, London.

Misuse of Drugs Regulations (1985) and amendments. HMSO, London.

Police and Criminal Evidence Act (1984). HMSO, London.

Preston A (1999). Green light for acid sales. *Druglink*, May/June, 7.

RPSGB (1998). *Report of the Working Party on Pharmaceutical Services for Drug Misusers: A Report to the Council of the Royal Pharmaceutical Society of Great Britain*. London.

RPSGB (2002). *Medicines, Ethics and Practice: A Guide for Pharmacists. 26th edition*, RPSGB, London.

Scottish Drugs Forum (1999). *Working with young drug users: Guidelines to developing policy*, Scottish Drugs Forum UN Convention on the Child (1989), Glasgow.

Strang J, Witton J, Hall W (2000a). Improving the quality of the cannabis debate: defining the different domains. *British Medical Journal*, 320, 108–110.

Strang J, Keaney F, Butterworth G, Noble A, Best D (2000b). Different forms of heroin and their relationship to cook-up techniques: Data on, and explanation of, use of lemon juice and other acids. *Substance Use and Misuse*, 36, 573–587.

10

The history and operation of pharmacy needle exchanges

Trish Shorrock

WHAT ARE NEEDLE AND SYRINGE EXCHANGES?

A needle and syringe exchange scheme is a facility whereby injecting drug users can obtain free needles and syringes, and return used ones for safe disposal, this service being available on a regular basis. Depending on where the exchange is based, additional services such as counselling about drug use, advice about safer injecting practices, etc., may also be provided.

WHY ARE NEEDLE AND SYRINGE EXCHANGES NEEDED?

Needle exchanges have been with us now in Britain since the mid-1980s, so it is clear that they do have a definite purpose. In brief they serve to limit the transmission of blood-borne infections such as HIV, and hepatitis B and C, which can be transmitted by the sharing of injecting equipment. The provision of free clean injecting equipment has been shown to be an effective strategy in reducing the sharing of injecting equipment (Donoghoe *et al.*, 1992).

In practice, however, needle exchanges often provide much more than just injecting equipment. They provide a safe and secure place to dispose of used injecting equipment, thus reducing the amount of used injecting equipment unsafely disposed of. They can also be a place where clients, who might otherwise be reluctant to approach services, go for general health or injecting advice which can lead to them accessing mainstream drug services for longer term help.

HOW DID NEEDLE AND SYRINGE EXCHANGES COME ABOUT?

The first syringe exchange schemes began in Britain in 1986 in Surrey, Peterborough, Dundee, Sheffield and Liverpool. Of these initial schemes, only one in Sheffield had any sort of pharmacy involvement (the others were all solely drug agency or hospital based). The syringe exchange in Sheffield was managed through the Sheffield Drug Abuse Service at the Royal Hallamshire Hospital and Sheffield Drugline. Clients came by either directly approaching these agencies or by going to a pharmacist who then referred them on. After counselling, the patients received a letter which they could take to one of six participating pharmacies, where they could buy and return used equipment.

This scheme then, was not in any way like the low threshold easy access pharmacy schemes of today, and it also merely enabled clients to buy equipment and return it, not receive it free. However, it did mark the initial involvement of pharmacies in the needle exchange process.

In 1987, a government-supported pilot experiment involving fifteen schemes began, influenced by the fact that there had emerged from Scotland strong evidence that the transmission of the HIV virus among injecting drug users (leading to extremely high rates of infection) had been facilitated by a shortage of syringes. There was a fear that this situation could be repeated elsewhere in Britain. Also, in the Netherlands distribution and exchange programmes had begun in 1984 (Buning, 1991) and in the mid-80s Norman Fowler, the then Secretary of State for Health (who had taken on AIDS as a special issue), made a well-publicised visit to Amsterdam to look at responses to AIDS. Short-term criteria for success involved investigating whether the programmes were established and operated as planned, whether they reached and retained potential clients and whether clients were helped to change their high risk behaviour.

The fifteen pilot schemes were based in twelve English and three Scottish towns/cities and included several of the schemes which had been operational since 1986. In addition to providing injecting equipment on an exchange basis, they were required to provide counselling for clients' drug problems, advice on safer sex and counselling on HIV testing. They were also to collect information on clients in order to collaborate with monitoring and evaluation requirements.

RESULTS OF THE PILOT SCHEME
The result of the initial evaluation study of the schemes was encouraging (Stimson *et al.*, 1988). It showed that the schemes reached potential clients in substantial numbers and that many of these were not presently in contact with drug services. Drug injectors attending exchanges were also helped to make important changes in their HIV risk behaviour. However, many clients did not remain in contact with the exchange and there was a high client turnover. Most clients (53%) who continued to attend lived nearby and travelled two miles or less to get to the exchange. The average age of attendance was 27.8 years and 78% of the clients were male (Donoghoe *et al.*, 1992). Thus it appeared that younger and/or female injectors were not using the service in significant numbers.

PHARMACY-BASED NEEDLE AND SYRINGE EXCHANGE SCHEMES AS THEY ARE TODAY: WHAT THEY ARE AND HOW THEY CAME ABOUT
In response to the findings of the initial evaluation of the pilot exchange schemes and to reach more injectors and groups either not previously reached or poorly reached (such as young people and female injectors), different models of service were developed. These were developed alongside the existing schemes based within hospitals or drug agencies, to complement them and increase accessibility. One of these approaches was pharmacy-based needle exchange schemes as we know them today.

The aim of pharmacy-based schemes, as with other schemes, was to help prevent the spread of the HIV virus by providing injecting drug users with free injecting equipment, condoms, health education information, and also providing a safe disposal service for used equipment. All these services were to be provided with a non-judgmental attitude and an awareness and respect for client confidentiality.

The Royal Pharmaceutical Society first issued guidelines for pharmacists taking part in needle and syringe exchange schemes in 1987 (RPSGB, 1987). This was a major change in policy for the profession, since in 1982, in an attempt to reduce the increasing number of injectors, the Royal Pharmaceutical Society of Great Britain had recommended that the sales of needles and syringes be restricted to "bona fide patients for therapeutic purposes only" (RPSGB, 1982). Fortunately, this recommendation was withdrawn in 1986 in view of the evidence about the spread of HIV by injecting drug use (RPSGB, 1986). Pharmacists from this point on were encouraged to reconsider their role in helping drug users and to give consideration to the sales of syringes. From there, it was just a small and obvious step for pharmacists to become involved fully in needle exchange schemes, and in 1989 the Pharmaceutical Society issued further, more detailed guidelines for pharmacists wishing to take part in such schemes (RPSGB, 1989).

WHY ARE PHARMACY SCHEMES A GOOD IDEA?

In 1993, in its report on HIV/AIDS and Drug Misuse, the Advisory Council on the Misuse of Drugs suggested that pharmacists should increase their level of involvement in needle exchange schemes (ACMD, 1993) and pharmacy needle exchange was praised by the Department of Health's effectiveness review of drug treatment (Department of Health, 1996).

Pharmacy-based needle exchange schemes offer many advantages. Firstly there are at present over 12,000 community pharmacies in the UK, which means that there is a large distribution of pharmacies in the areas where people live, and approximately 20% of pharmacies in England and Wales provide this service (Sheridan *et al.*, 1996). Even if only a proportion are involved in needle exchange schemes, it still greatly increases the accessibility for clients. Furthermore, most community pharmacies are open for longer hours than drug agencies and also on additional days (for example, week-ends).

Secondly, entering a community pharmacy has no stigma attached to it, which may be especially important for certain clients. For example, women with children may be quite reluctant to enter a drug agency, because of fears about losing custody should anyone see them and thus find out about their drug use.

Finally, the pharmacists themselves are there as a source of health information and advice and, importantly, are available for consultation without an appointment. Hopefully, all pharmacists participating in needle exchange schemes will also be both tactful and non-judgmental, and fully aware of confidentiality requirements.

It should be emphasised at this point that whilst pharmacy schemes offer many advantages over agency schemes, they are in no way in "competition" with them. There are many things which agency-based needle exchange schemes offer, which pharmacy schemes cannot – for example, in-depth counselling, inspection of injection sites etc. Pharmacy schemes are there to complement agency schemes and should work closely with the local drug agency. There are times when it will be appropriate to refer a client to the local drug agency, but it is obviously not appropriate to do this in every case. It has been postulated that pharmacists in many instances will see a largely different population of clients to that seen in agencies. Evidence of this was shown by a survey of over 200 clients of a pharmacy-based needle exchange scheme, which showed that 49% were not presently in touch with a GP, drug agency or other health professional about their drug use (Anthony *et al.*, 1995). Examples of these clients can include younger drug users in an early phase of their drug using career. Such clients may not yet have encountered any problems associated with their drug use and merely require a low threshold service which gives them easy access to clean injecting equipment and a place to dispose of used equipment safely. Obviously, trying to automatically refer such clients to an agency would be counter-productive. Pharmacists, as healthcare professionals, must use their judgement about when referral to an agency is necessary. Thus, the pharmacy can act as a potential point of entry for referral to other helping agencies.

HOW ARE SCHEMES OPERATED?

In 1992, the Centre for Research on Drug and Health Behaviour published an overview of syringe exchanges in England. It stated that "the syringe exchange strat-egy developed from a centralised government-led and funded initiative to one in which individual exchanges have a great deal of local autonomy…such a develop-ment has facilitated local solutions to local problems" (Donoghoe *et al.*, 1992). The latter statement, whilst referring to needle exchange schemes in general, is especially relevant to pharmacy schemes. Whilst the Royal Pharmaceutical Society of Great Britain has regularly updated its guidelines for pharmacists who take part in needle exchange schemes (RPSGB, 1993, 2001), the overall running of the schemes along with issues about equipment supplied, returns policies, records kept, etc., varies con-siderably. Even the issue about who co-ordinates pharmacy-based schemes is not clear cut. In some instances, it is someone from the local drug agency, in others it may be someone from the Primary Care Trust (PCT), or even a member of a health pro-motion department. Because of such wide differences it is difficult to give a specific overview of how a scheme operates. However, areas such as equipment, registration, etc., will be broadly discussed below. If pharmacists wish to join their local needle exchange scheme they should find out who the co-ordinator is (calling the local drug agency or the PCT should provide this information). The local co-ordinator will advise as to the protocol operating in that area.

WHAT EQUIPMENT IS SUPPLIED?

Many schemes operate on a pack system with a number of particular needles and syringes provided in a ready made up pack containing different sizes of needles and syringes. For example, many schemes provide 1 ml packs, 2 ml packs and 5 ml packs containing 1 ml, 2 ml and 5 ml syringes respectively. Different sized syringes are used according to both personal preferences of clients and also relating to the drug used (for example, steroid users tend to inject larger amounts of drug intramuscularly than heroin users do intravenously). Different sized needles may also be included, for example, whilst smaller "orange" needles (gauge 0.5 mm, length 16 mm) are fine for injecting into veins, steroid users who inject into muscle would need a longer, thicker "green" needle (gauge 0.8 mm, length 40 mm). Packs also usually contain other items such as sterile swabs, condoms and leaflets containing advice about safer injecting. However, not all schemes operate this "pack" system; some operate what is known as a "pick and mix" system whereby a variety of loose needles, syringes, swabs, etc., are kept by the pharmacy and clients select what equipment they want individually.

HOW MUCH EQUIPMENT SHOULD BE GIVEN OUT?

Again, this will vary according to local protocol, although in many, whilst the protocol provides pharmacists with some guidance, there is flexibility for the pharmacist to make their own decision. It is quite likely that clients may on occasions want to take injecting equipment for other people as well as themselves. Encouraging their fellow injectors to register as well is considered a good idea, but in some cases people may be reluctant to do so, or it may be difficult for them to get to the scheme (often a problem in rural areas). In these cases it is imperative to remember the principles behind harm minimisation i.e. that our first goal in working with drug-using clients must be to help them avoid acquiring or transmitting blood-borne viruses such as HIV and hepatitis B and C. Refusal to issue extra equipment could lead to sharing of needles and syringes with the inherent risk of transmitting just such blood-borne diseases.

WHAT ABOUT DISPOSAL OF USED EQUIPMENT?

Most schemes, when supplying injecting equipment, provide a small-sized individual sharps container for disposal of used equipment (examples being Intercobra tubes). These can then be returned to the pharmacy when full. The usual procedure is that a client places these individual sharps containers in a larger sharps bin kept by the pharmacist. This means that no member of staff ever touches loose needles and syringes. As with the injecting equipment, the disposal equipment should be provided by the scheme co-ordinator, who should also arrange for collection and incineration of full sharps containers.

HOW IS REGISTRATION/RECORD KEEPING DEALT WITH?

With all schemes, inevitably there is some paperwork. In most areas when clients first approach a scheme, they are asked to register, giving basic details such as their initials or name, date of birth and their approximate area of residence (e.g. first three letters of postcode if known). This is not to try to identify the client, but to monitor who uses the scheme, and identify areas where schemes are needed, but not currently operating. It is important to explain to clients why the information is being asked for and to reassure them as to the confidential nature of the scheme. The identity of people using the scheme should not be revealed to anyone (including GPs, or even the police) without first discussing it with the scheme co-ordinator).

In certain schemes after registering, clients receive a numbered key fob, which they produce each time they use a pharmacy in the scheme. In other areas this approach has proved less popular and individual record sheets for each client are kept and used whenever the client presents to a particular shop (using initials and dates of birth usually prevents double counting if clients use more than one shop). Pharmacists also generally record on each transaction the amount and type of equipment issued and any returns made.

SHOULD EQUIPMENT ONLY BE SUPPLIED ON A ONE-FOR-ONE EXCHANGE BASIS?

In general, the idea behind schemes was that they were "exchange schemes" which does imply a one-for-one exchange policy. However, in reality most pharmacists have recognised the impracticality of this and in order to ensure the reduction of transmission of blood-borne viruses have become more flexible, and do not insist on a one-for-one exchange in every instance, whilst still, however, strongly encouraging returns. A good pointer is to ask those clients who frequently don't return where they are disposing of their used equipment. In some cases they may be returning to the drug agency. Policies do differ, however, from area to area and the local scheme co-ordinator can clarify what their protocol denotes.

WHAT ABOUT TRAINING?

Training for pharmacists and pharmacy staff should be provided by scheme co-ordinators. The extent of this training may vary from whole training days/evenings to the provision of detailed training/information packs for the pharmacists and staff to work through in their own time. Areas covered include general information about substance misuse, safer injecting and information about blood-borne infections. There must also be a protocol which describes the service provided and which details also the action to be taken in the case of accidents such as the spillage of infected blood or syringes. It is also worthwhile noting that there is now much more information about substance misuse specially tailored for pharmacists, both in book form and in the form of nationally available distance-learning packs.

PAYMENT

Again, payment systems vary widely, but most allow for a modest retainer fee for participating pharmacists each year, with additional payments based on the number of packs given out and also possibly the number of clients seen (i.e. payment scales should reflect the amount of time pharmacists spend in connection with the scheme).

SHOULD ONLY THE PHARMACIST PERFORM THE EXCHANGE?

Whilst this was previously insisted upon, this is now no longer the case in the UK. The RPSGB's code of ethics in 1997, referring to needle exchange services, stated that "supplies of syringes and needles must be made by the pharmacist or appropriately trained staff" (RPSGB, 1997a). This clearly implies that staff in addition to pharmacists may be suitably trained and therefore involved in needle exchange procedures.

WHAT ABOUT SUPPLIES TO UNDER-16s?

This is a difficult area and one which has been subject to much debate and confusion. In April 1991 the RPSGB issued the following statement:

> "that no objection be made to the inclusion of drug abusers under the age of 16 years in needle and syringe exchange schemes. The decision was made in recognition of the fact that the transmission of HIV infection bore no relation to the age of the user" (RPSGB, 1991).

Hence is seemed quite clear that their was no objection to pharmacists potentially supplying injecting equipment to under-16s, should they deem it necessary in terms of harm minimisation.

However, in 1993 new council guidelines were issued which, under the heading "Supplies to Children" stated that "Extra caution should be exercised in supplies to children under the age of 16 years. Such clients should normally be referred to a specialist agency" (RPSGB, 1993).

Whilst undoubtedly sensible advice, this has left some pharmacists with a particular dilemma. What if they know a young person is injecting, but the young person refuses to go to a drug agency? Even within drug agencies the issue about supplying to under 16s is an issue. Much has been gleaned from the case of Gillick v Norfolk and Wisbech AHA and the DHSS, which involved giving contraceptive advice and treatment to under-16s without parental consent. The judges in that case effectively delegated responsibility for decisions about under-16s to professionals (in that case doctors) better qualified than they to deal with cases on an individual basis. Basically in order to be in line with the 1989 Children Act, which states that the welfare of the child is paramount, workers must satisfy themselves that the young person will benefit from receiving advice, treatment or both, be it with or without parental consent.

Where this leaves pharmacists then, is unclear, and it is best once again to discuss such issues with the local scheme co-ordinator. For more information on this issue and other relating to services for under-16s, see Chapter 9.

SUPPLIES OF CITRIC ACID, AND OTHER INJECTING PARAPHERNALIA

Pharmacists who participate in needle exchange schemes may well be asked by clients using the scheme to sell them citric acid. Citric acid is, in fact, used by heroin injectors to help dissolve some types of street heroin in water. Other types of acid used to dissolve heroin have in the past included vinegar or lemon juice, but this itself can be contaminated and has led in the past to fungal infections of the eye (Hay, 1986; Strang *et al.*, 2001). Selling citric acid, then, could be thought of as a harm minimisation approach, since it reduces the possibility of damage to a client's veins. However, to sell citric acid when it is known that it will be used in connection with substance misuse is currently an offence under Section 9a of the Misuse of Drugs Act, as it is counted as paraphernalia.

Other items which are included as paraphernalia are spoons, filters, tourniquets and also sterile wipes. Interestingly, most needle exchange schemes (including pharmacies) have given out sterile wipes since their start, but technically this is not legal. However, in the case of citric acid, the position of the pharmacist is an awkward one. Whilst it appears very unlikely that a prosecution about such a sale would ever occur, to sell citric acid to a client does contravene the law as it stands at present. A recent working party of the RPSGB, set up to look at services for drug misusers, recommended amongst other things that "the Misuse of Drugs Act 1971 should be amended to allow clients to supply citric acid, water for injections, filters, tourniquets and swabs...supplying paraphernalia through pharmacies would provide an opportunity for discussing other aspects of safe injecting techniques and lifestyle changes." (RPSGB, 1998). However, whether this report will be acted upon by the Department of Health and the Home Office remains to be seen.

A possible way forward in the meantime has been illustrated in Dorset, where the local drug service has obtained reassurance from both the Police and the Crown

Prosecution Service that neither investigation nor prosecution were being considered despite the fact that they were contravening section 9a of the Misuse of Drugs Act. The rationale behind this being that the law was never intended to prevent harm reduction measures. In response to the Dorset situation, the Royal Pharmaceutical Society of Great Britain confirmed that, in the absence of a prosecution (or a wider charge of misconduct), it would not discipline members who break section 9a of the Misuse of Drugs Act (Preston, 1999).

In Scotland, the advice from the Lord Advocate via the Regional Procurators Fiscal is that pharmacists involved in needle exchanges in Greater Glasgow and Lanarkshire can supply citric acid as part of a harm reduction initiative (Scottish Executive, 2001).

BEHAVIOUR OF CLIENTS

This is often an area of concern for pharmacists who are considering taking part in a needle and syringe exchange scheme. In fact, pharmacists are not alone in having reservations about providing services for drug users. Amongst GPs negative attitudes are also not uncommon (Greenwood, 1992). There is no doubt that some drug using clients either picking up prescriptions or using needle exchange schemes can occasionally be difficult, but on the whole most pharmacists do not find their worst fears about excessive shoplifting, violence, etc., are realised. There is also evidence to indicate that those displaying a negative attitude to drug users are more likely to experience negative behaviour such as shoplifting and abuse (Matheson, 1998). On the whole, most pharmacists operating schemes who use a friendly and non-judgmental attitude appear to encounter reasonably few problems, as the majority of clients do appreciate the service and behave accordingly. If this was not the case, it is unlikely that any such schemes would still be taking place.

SALES OF NEEDLES AND SYRINGES

For those pharmacists not participating in a needle exchange scheme there used to be the option of selling needles and syringes to drug users on request. However, in November 1997 the RPSGB issued a council statement that "only in exceptional circumstances should pharmacists supply clean injecting equipment for drug misusers if the pharmacy has no arrangements for taking back contaminated equipment." (RPSGB, 1997b). It is unclear what exactly would constitute an "exceptional circumstance", but it means that it is even more essential for pharmacists not participating in schemes to know where the nearest needle exchange schemes are. Those receiving frequent requests for sales should possibly consider joining a scheme or asking the local scheme organiser if they can provide a sharps container and arrange for its collection and incineration when full.

CONFIDENTIALITY

One of the major factors which is essential for the success of syringe exchange schemes is that are promoted as, and seen to be completely confidential. This means that unless the client has given their consent, information about their use of the scheme should not be disclosed to anyone, not even their GP or drug worker.

Pharmacists participating in needle exchange schemes sometimes feel themselves to have an ethical dilemma when a methadone patient requests injecting equipment. In this instance the temptation might be to inform the presciber; however the entire pharmacy needle and syringe exchange scheme would be jeopardised by no longer being considered confidential. Also partners and friends often collect for each other.

Not informing prescribers about a client's use of needle exchange services does not contravene the Royal Pharmaceutical Society's Code of Ethics as the code states that "the public expects pharmacists and their staff to respect and protect confidentiality. This duty extends to any information relating to an individual which pharmacists or their staff acquire in the course of their professional activities" (RPSGB, 2001).

There are obviously some expectations for example:

- where disclosure of the information is to a person or body empowered by statute to require such a disclosure;
- where necessary to prevent serious injury or damage to the health of the patient or a third party or to public health.

HOW ARE SCHEMES ADVERTISED?

Advertising for pharmacy needle exchange schemes tends to be very low-key. Participating pharmacies tend to display a recognised window sticker in their pharmacy window. In most cases this is the now nationally recognised two arrow logo, although a small number of local schemes may have their own logo as well. The two arrow logo is extremely discreet and has no significance to people unaware of the scheme. It is extremely important to have a nationally recognised logo, as drug users, like the rest of us, do not always stay in the same place and need to be able to identify participating pharmacies easily, if they do visit another area. Some schemes also include leaflets with the injecting equipment they give out, which detail other local participating pharmacies. However, the most effective source of advertising appears to be word of mouth, with clients hearing about schemes from other clients.

FIFTEEN YEARS ON: IS THE TARGET STILL THE SAME?

In the fifteen years since needle and syringe exchanges were first set up, many things have changed. For example, awareness of other blood-borne infections as well as HIV has increased considerably. Hepatitis B and even more importantly, hepatitis C, have been recognised as real dangers for injecting drug users. There are estimates that approximately 60% of injecting drug users have hepatitis C (Waller and Holmes, 1995; Majid *et al.*, 1995) with some estimates being as high as almost 80% (Best *et al.*, 1999), and therefore it has in many ways become as much, if not more, of a focus than HIV and AIDS.

Also in the years since exchanges were first established an awareness and understanding of clients such as steroid users has developed. In 1991, Royal Pharmaceutical Society of Great Britain accepted a recommendation of the Ethics Committee that "no objection should be made to the inclusion of users of anabolic steroids in schemes for the supply or exchange of hypodermic needles and syringes" (RPSGB, 1991). Interestingly this appears to imply that up till this point steroid users should not have been allowed to obtain injecting equipment from pharmacy-based schemes, although whether they were in any way excluded prior to this time is very much in doubt. Most needle and syringe exchange schemes now know that other groups such as steroid users may require different injecting equipment to other injecting drug users, and need to be reached/targeted using a different approach.

FIFTEEN YEARS ON: HAS NEEDLE AND SYRINGE EXCHANGE WORKED?

With regard to the reductions in syringe sharing behaviour, several reports point to a reduction in this and, to a great extent, in most contexts safer injecting practices have become standard. That is not to say, however, that syringe or paraphernalia sharing has been eliminated. Indeed, it is foolish to be complacent, particularly in the light of recent evidence that hepatitis C infection has been identified in significant numbers of injectors who commenced injecting after the establishment of needle and syringe exchange facilities (van Beek *et al.*, 1998). However, estimates show that in England (outside London) the HIV prevalence rate amongst injectors continues to be less than 1% (Unlinked Anonymous HIV and Screening Surveys Group, 1995) and the rate within London is much lower than in other cities such as New York, Paris, Rome and Madrid, where injecting drug use is also prevalent (Ball *et al.*, 1995). The previously high rate in Edinburgh of 50% has also been reduced to about 20% (Public Health Laboratory Service, 1997).

No evidence has shown that needle exchange programmes increase the amount of drug use by needle exchange clients or in the wider community. In Amsterdam, annual capture-recapture studies of "hard" drug users showed their numbers to be stable, the mean age of this population to be increasing and the proportion of under-22s to be declining (Buning, 1991). Thus it appears that the investment in prevention has paid off and should be continued, in order that the present situation be maintained.

CONCLUSION
Problem areas and the way forward for pharmacies

It seems clear that needle and syringe exchange programmes have been effective to a large extent in changing injecting risk behaviours. However, where they have been less successful is in changing the sexual behaviour of injecting drug users (Donoghoe *et al.*, 1992). Injecting drug users are seen in most studies to show levels of condom use comparable with the heterosexual population as a whole, and there appears to have been a lack of any notable sexual behaviour change amongst drug injectors.

It is therefore important that pharmacists remember that as well as advice about injecting practice and drug-related dangers, advice about contraception, safer sex, etc., may be sought by needle exchange clients. The displaying of appropriate literature might also be a way of spreading the message about contraception, sexual health and safer sex. A friendly, non-judgmental attitude to pregnant drug users may also encourage them to seek health advice and receive appropriate treatment and ante-natal care.

Another area of great concern is the potential risk of acquiring blood-borne infections through the shared use of paraphernalia such as water, spoons, cups, filters, etc. This is of particular concern in the case of hepatitis B and C, which are much more robust viruses than the HIV virus. With rates of infection of injecting drug users with hepatitis C being estimated as being at least 60% (Waller and Holmes, 1995; Best *et al.*, 1999), this is a cause for great concern. Once again, pharmacists need to be aware of these issues and be on hand to provide appropriate advice to injecting drug users that "sharing" includes not just needles and syringes.

Another vital opportunity for pharmacists involves the role of promoting good general health and providing general health advice to drug users who, in many instances, see no other health professionals at all. Pharmacists in this instance can be vitally important, and once again may eventually be the referral point to another helping service such as a GP.

Finally, pharmacists can be rightly proud of the role they have played in harm minimisation approaches to date. The idea of needle and syringe exchange schemes is a typical example of a "knowledge and means approach" to behaviour change. That is, it helps to provide individuals with knowledge about risk and risk behaviour, along with providing them with the means to make changes in it (e.g. by providing them with sterile injecting equipment). Hopefully, this pragmatic approach will continue, with pharmacists taking their proper place working alongside drug agencies to provide a useful and comprehensive network of services for clients with drug misuse problems and health needs.

REFERENCES

Advisory Council on the Misuse of Drugs (1993). *AIDS and Drug Misuse Update*. Department of Health, London.

Anthony R, Shorrock PJ, Christie M (1995). *Pharmacy-based Needle and Syringe Exchange Schemes: An Evaluation within Trent Region*. Nepenthe Press, Leicestershire Community Drug and Alcohol Services.

Ball A, Des Jarlais D, Donoghoe MC (1995). *Multi-centre study on drug injecting and risk of HIV infection: A report prepared on behalf of the international collaborative group for the World Health Organisation Programme on Substance Abuse*. Geneva, World Health Organisation.

Best D, Noble A, Finch E, Gossop M, Sidwell C, Strang J (1999). Accuracy of perceptions of hepatitis B and C Status: cross sectional investigation of opiate addicts in treatment. *British Medical Journal*, 319, 290–291.

Buning EEC (1991). Effects of Amsterdam needle and syringe exchange. *International Journal of Addiction*, 26, 1303–1311.

Department of Health (1996). *The Task Force to review services for drug misusers – report of an independent review of drug treatment services in England*, HMSO, London.

Donoghoe MC, Stimson CV, Dolan KA (1992). *Syringe Exchange in England: An Overview*. The Centre for Research on Drugs and Health Behaviour, London.

Greenwood J (1992). Unpopular Patients: GPs' attitudes to drug users. *Druglink*, July/August, 8–10.

Hay RJ (1986). Systemic candidiasis in heroin addicts. *British Medical Journal*, 292, 1096.

Majid A, Holmes R, Desselberger U, Simmonds P, McKee TA (1995). Molecular epidemiology of hepatitis C infection among intravenous drug users in rural communities. *Journal of Medical Virololgy*, 46, 48–51.

Matheson C (1998). Views of illicit drug users on their treatment and behaviour in Scottish community pharmacies: implications for the harm reduction strategy. *Health Education Journal*, 57, 31–41.

Preston A (1999). Green light for acid sales. *Druglink*, May/June, 7.

Public Health Laboratory Service (1997). *The epidemiology of HIV infection and AIDS. Communicable Diseases Review Vol. 7 Review No. 9*. Public Health Laboratory Service, Communicable Diseases Surveillance Centre, London.

Royal Pharmaceutical Society of Great Britain (RPSGB) (1982). Council Statement, Sale of syringes. *Pharmaceutical Journal*, 228, 692.

Royal Pharmaceutical Society of Great Britain (RPSGB) (1986). Council Statement, Sale of hypodermic syringes and needles. *Pharmaceutical Journal*, 236, 205.

Royal Pharmaceutical Society of Great Britain (RPSGB) (1987). Council Guidance. Guidelines for pharmacists involved in schemes to supply clean syringes and needles to addicts. *Pharmaceutical Journal*, 238, 481.

Royal Pharmaceutical Society of Great Britain (RPSGB) (1989). Council Guidance. Guidelines for pharmacists involved in schemes to supply clean syringes and needles to addicts. *Pharmaceutical Journal*, 242, 176.

Royal Pharmaceutical Society of Great Britain (RPSGB) (1991). Council Guidance. Needle and syringe supply. *Pharmaceutical Journal*, 246, 488.

Royal Pharmaceutical Society of Great Britain (RPSGB) (1993). Council Guidance. Syringe and needle supply. *Pharmaceutical Journal*, 251, 20.

Royal Pharmaceutical Society of Great Britain (RPSGB) (1997a). Standards for pharmacists providing needle and syringe exchange schemes. *Pharmaceutical Journal*, 259, 963–964.

Royal Pharmaceutical Society of Great Britain (RPSGB) (1997b). Needles for drug misusers. *Pharmaceutical Journal*, 259, 803.

Royal Pharmaceutical Society of Great Britain Working Party (1998). *Pharmaceutical Services for Drug Misusers. Report on pharmaceutical services for drug misusers.* RPSGB, London.

Royal Pharmaceutical Society of Great Britain (RPSGB) (2001). *Medicines, Ethics and Practice: a guide for pharmacists, 25th edition,* RPSGB, London.

Scottish Executive, Substance Misuse Division (2001). *Guidance on Drug Misuse Services and Prevention of Blood-Borne Viruses.* Annex E. Scottish Executive, Edinburgh.

Sheridan J, Lovell S, Parsons J, Turnbull J, Stimson GV, Strang J (2000). Pharmacy-based needle exchange (PBNX) schemes in South-East London. *Addiction*, 95, 1551–1560.

Sheridan J, Strang J, Barber N, Glanz A (1996). Role of community pharmacies in relation to HIV prevention and drug misuse: findings from the 1995 national survey in England and Wales. *British Medical Journal*, 313, 272–274.

Stimson GV *et al.* (1988). Syringe Exchange Schemes for drug users in England and Scotland. *British Medical Journal*, 296, 1717–1719.

Strang J, Keaney F, Butterworth G, Noble A, Best D (2001). Different forms of heroin and their relationship to cook-up techniques: data on, and explanation of, use of lemon juice and other acids. *Substance Use and Misuse*, 36, 573–587.

Unlinked Anonymous HIV Surveys Steering Group (1995). *Unlinked anonymous HIV prevalence Monitoring Programme: England and Wales.* Department of Health, London.

van Beek I, Dwyer R, Dore G, Luo K, Kaldor JM (1998). Infection with HIV and hepatitis C virus among injecting drug users in a prevention setting: retrospective cohort study. *British Medical Journal,* 317, 433–437.

Waller T, Holmes R (1995). The Sleeping Giant Wakes. Hepatitis C: Scale and impact in Britain. *Druglink,* September/October 8–11.

11

Professional conflicts for the front-line pharmacist

Janie Sheridan, Gihan Butterworth and Christine Glover

This chapter will examine some practical issues that relate to providing services for drug users in a community pharmacy setting. In providing services, pharmacists may on occasions, find themselves in positions where they are either having to deal with a difficult or threatening situation, or where they are faced with an ethical or professional dilemma. The latter are dealt with in Chapter 9, so in this chapter there will be a focus on more practical issues such as how to manage patient numbers, inappropriate requests for methadone supply and disruptive behaviour.

It is important to remember that problems faced by pharmacists can be related to any of their patients or customers – and that it is not just drug users who may be the source of problems. In addition, it is noteworthy that it is rare for drug users to cause serious problems for pharmacists, a case of a minority spoiling it for the majority. Indeed, around half of the community pharmacies in England and Wales dispense prescriptions for the management of drug misuse and almost one fifth are involved in needle exchange (Sheridan *et al.*, 1996). We may therefore assume that for the majority of those pharmacies, services are provided in a normal fashion with little disruption to the pharmacy, the staff and other customers.

Research carried out in the mid 1990s, which looked at pharmacies in London, found that pharmacists and their staff had indeed experienced threats of violence or violent attacks; however, such events were not committed solely by drug users, but by a wide variety of "customers" (Smith and Weidner, 1996a,b). The authors surmise that simply being a retail environment means the community pharmacy is an obvious place for crime to occur.

In looking at some of the issues around providing services to drug users, and indeed to all our patients and customers, it may be timely to remind ourselves exactly what kind of services we are aiming to offer. Thus, a number of issues can be examined such as the attitudes of staff and pharmacists, some of the problems that may be encountered and how to manage them, and how to deal with conflicts in the pharmacy.

PHARMACIST AND STAFF ATTITUDES
Of all the potential problems, pharmacist and staff attitudes are possibly the most crucial. For example, research has shown that pharmacists often have negative attitudes

towards drug users (Sheridan *et al.*, 1997; Matheson *et al.*, 1999) and that drug users are aware of being stigmatised (Matheson, 1998) and will be sensitive to any treatment they regard as judgmental.

Drug misuse and drug misusers are issues within society and most people are aware of the problem. However, the extent of an individual's understanding about drug misuse will be based on a number of things such as personal experience, their exposure to media coverage with varying degrees of accuracy or sensationalism, and in the case of pharmacists and their staff, professional contact with drug misusers. At a personal level, each individual is entitled to his or her own view, but in professional circumstances, it would be reasonable to expect practitioners who undertake any service provision for this patient group, to have a "professional" and non-judgmental approach. Such an approach will have a positive impact on any potential problems that may arise as a result of offering this service.

It is also clear that people who have experienced unpleasant or even dangerous events involving drug users are less likely to hold particularly positive attitudes. It is therefore important for pharmacists to be aware of their own and their staff's feelings and concerns, and to try and deal with them in a positive way.

In addition, pharmacy staff should be aware of their roles and the limitations of these roles, which should also be understood by patients. Staff (including pharmacists) should be firm, fair and consistent, although some degree of flexibility should be allowed.

While a significant proportion of community pharmacists will be involved in the care of drug users, they may lack an in-depth understanding of the nature of substance misuse and treatments available. Training and education are essential so that service providers understand the philosophy of harm reduction surrounding the decision to treat a patient. These training requirements need to go beyond the "pharmaceutical" aspects of methadone. From this point of view, multi-professional training will encourage the sharing of experiences and help to iron out problems. Training for pharmacists and their staff should also cover more practical aspects of service provision such as how to diffuse difficult situations and how to deal with aggression. Training should be provided to pharmacy assistants and to the staff who are responsible for the day-to-day running of services such as needle exchange, who are often the first port of call for drug users.

WHAT TYPES OF PROBLEMS ARE LIKELY TO OCCUR AND HOW TO MANAGE THEM?
Confidentiality
The management of drug misuse may include the use of a multi-disciplinary, multi-agency approach. Indeed, the new Departments of Health clinical guidelines (1999) recommend a shared care approach. This will therefore have an impact on the pharmacist who may have to communicate and collaborate with a number of different individuals. In general, most pharmacists will be used to communicating with the prescribing doctor, particularly in relation to drug misusers, and often only when there is a specific prescription-related problem. However, with the shared-care, multi-disciplinary, approach to treatment for this patient group, they may be required to feed back information about a patient's well-being on a more regular and formalised basis to other members of the team, within the bounds of confidentiality, and care for that individual patient.

Because much drug misuse involves the use of illicit substances such as heroin or cocaine, drug users tend to be particularly concerned about who will have access to information about them and their activities. They may also be concerned that the prescriber may find out that they use the needle exchange, when they are being prescribed oral methadone. Or they may be concerned about the police finding out that they are a drug user. From this point of view it is important for pharmacists to have a clear understanding about the issues surrounding confidentiality and with whom they are allowed to communicate what. Such issues are covered in Chapter 9.

To avoid conflict around the area of confidentiality, the pharmacist should be clear with the patient, from the start, what information will be shared with whom. In some cases it may be wise to obtain written consent from the patient to disclose such information. This should be kept fairly general so as to cover most probable situations.

Privacy

Another area of particular importance to drug users is that of privacy. Some of the services provided by pharmacists to drug users involve patients participating in certain activities such as drinking methadone in the pharmacy or exchanging used for clean injecting equipment. In such instances it is important to remember that they may not want to have those actions observed and should be afforded the privacy required. This can be done in a number of ways, the simplest being by informing the patient when the pharmacy is likely to be the least busy. Additionally, pharmacists may wish to install a screened area from which they can provide a more confidential service to drug users and other customers. It is probably better, in terms of safety and security, not have this screened off area as a separate room.

Patient behaviour and patient demands

Many pharmacists cite patient behaviour as a reason for not providing services to this group (Sheridan *et al.*, 1996, 1997) and indeed drug users themselves are aware of the negative behaviour of their peers (Matheson, 1998). The majority of drug users behave as normally as other patients or customers. However, in a minority of cases, a patient's lifestyle can be chaotic and difficult and they may present this way at the pharmacy. Their language, in such instances, is often "less polite" and may be overtly aggressive, making interactions more difficult. However, it is important to keep this in perspective and to remember that community pharmacists will also experience angry and irrational behaviour from a minority of their non-drug-using patients and customers from time to time.

Some drug users are accustomed to being instantly rewarded through the effects of drug taking. They may expect instant attention in the pharmacy and thus may become irritable or frustrated at having to wait in a queue. Some may, quite reason-ably, expect their prescription to be ready for collection if they arrive at the same time each day. It is important to remember many feel stigmatised at having to pick up their prescription daily. Maybe, as mentioned previously, this is because they are sensitive to discrimination. At the start of treatment, it may be possible to negotiate with the patient, a time when the pharmacy is quiet or a time when their medication will be ready for collection. This should help build a positive relationship and minimise any conflicts around this issue.

Intoxication/safety issues

Oral methadone, unlike injected heroin, given daily, in constant doses, does not produce a profound euphoria. Furthermore, with the development of tolerance, drowsiness caused by methadone is unlikely. However illicit use "on top" of prescribed medication is not uncommon and some patients may behave inconsistently, due to the effects of the other drugs they use. The use of certain drugs is particularly associated with aggressive behaviour – for example, crack cocaine, amphetamine and alcohol. Conversely opiate users tend to be calmer and often sedated or intoxicated.

An intoxicated patient will present the pharmacist (and pharmacy staff) with a number of potential conflict issues. The interaction between opiates and other CNS depressants is a potentially fatal one and there will be occasions when the pharmacist will have to use their professional judgement to decide whether to supply or administer medication to an intoxicated patient. This ethical issue is discussed further in Chapter 9.

It may be difficult to assess whether a patient is intoxicated from only visual observations in a community pharmacy setting. If in doubt, it may be appropriate to send the patient back to the prescribing doctor, clinic or drug team for further assessment. A decision not to dispense may result in a patient becoming very hostile and/or aggressive, even if they have previously signed a patient agreement stating that they will not be dispensed to in such circumstances. As already mentioned, some drugs of misuse, including alcohol, are associated with aggressive behaviour and this may increase the possibility of a conflict situation.

A similar situation may arise if a patient has missed several doses of medication and it is unsafe to dispense because the patient's tolerance may have reduced. Once again a patient may need to be assessed by the prescribing doctors and the dose may need to be altered. A methadone patient in a state of withdrawal will be feeling unwell and may become difficult and hostile if a pharmacist refuses to dispense.

Of course, not all drug misusers will react in an aggressive manner in instances such as those described above. However, it is important that all pharmacy staff are aware of the possibility of such situations arising and are able to deal with them in an appropriate manner.

Prescription-related problems

All sorts of problems can occur which relate to the prescription itself. Some of these are common to all prescriptions, such as a drug being out of stock or the prescription being out of date or not signed by the doctor. Some problems are specific to Controlled Drug [CD] prescriptions, due to the nature of the strict regulations concerning the way the prescription must be written, which is absolute in the UK, allowing no room for clinical or professional judgement in this case. With regard to methadone prescriptions and other CD prescriptions for instalment dispensing, further problems may occur when there is a Public Holiday and the prescription has not been written to cover advance instalments for the days on which the pharmacy is closed.

The current Misuse of Drugs Regulations are so specific that a pharmacist is likely to come across many prescriptions that he/she cannot dispense legally and these issues are covered in more detail in Chapter 9. Refusing to dispense such a prescription can result in a patient becoming very upset and aggressive because they may perceive the pharmacist as being difficult over trivial problems and unreasonably withholding their medication.

It is important to remember that not all drug misusers will react in this way. Most will be reasonable and understand the situation, and many of the rest will respond to a firm, fair and consistent approach. It will help if the patient feels that their concerns are being listened to and that the pharmacist is trying to find a solution. Expressing empathy may also help.

Problems may be reduced if the pharmacist checks the prescription carefully on presentation. If there is a problem, there may be time to find a solution, before there is an interruption of supply of the patient's medication.

Methadone patients may also create problems by either requesting instalments of methadone to be dispensed in advance or asking to collect doses they have failed to collect in the past. They may also turn up for their methadone when a prescription has run out. The Misuse of Drugs Regulations relating to instalment dispensing state clearly that instalments can only be supplied on the day stated on the prescription. Patients requesting pharmacists to vary their supply from what is requested on the prescription must be met with a refusal. Such a refusal may result in confrontation. This may be minimised by explaining the rules of instalment dispensing to the patient at the start of treatment.

A major area of concern when looking at legal issues is that of prescription fraud. If the pharmacist accuses the patient of fraud face-to-face, it may precipitate violence. The pharmacist may not feel that they are in a position to effectively deal with possible aggressive behaviour. There may not be adequate numbers of staff, or members of the public may be put at risk. In this situation it would be advisable to make an excuse not to dispense, for example to say that an item is out of stock, and ask the patient to return later to allow time to obtain back-up and to provide time to check with the prescribing doctor or contact the police, if appropriate. It would be helpful to the police to retain the prescription; however if the patient insists on taking back the prescription, the pharmacist should not refuse to do so if this puts any staff in danger. It may be useful to take a photocopy of the prescription in circumstances where this is possible. Details of the prescription, including prescription serial number, and a description of the patient are often very helpful. The pharmacist can also mark the prescription with the "pharmacy stamp" to indicate to other pharmacists that the prescription should not be dispensed. Careful handling of the situation is vital, as the patient, and the potential for violence, may be unknown to the pharmacist. Staff should be encouraged to make a note of the description of the person.

Requests for injecting paraphernalia

Pharmacists are allowed to provide injecting drug users with clean injecting equipment and a means of safely disposing of used equipment. Many drug users believe that pharmacists will also be able to supply them with other "paraphernalia" associated with injecting drugs. These are items such as tourniquets, filters, citric and ascorbic acid (used to aid the dissolution of "black-market" heroin in the UK), and sterile water for injection (which is a "prescription only medicine" in the UK). However, the restrictions of Section 9A of the Misuse of Drugs Act currently prohibits their supply for this purpose. Within the broader context of harm reduction, it seems illogical to withhold such items. Indeed, many non-pharmacy needle and syringe exchange schemes supply citric acid, filters and tourniquets (albeit at odds with the law), yet pharmacies are unable to do so. Prescribers and drug agencies may not be aware of this and may direct patients wishing to obtain injecting paraphernalia to pharmacy needle and syringe exchanges.

Requests for sales of such items, when met with a refusal from pharmacy staff, may precipitate an unpleasant incident. The patient may be unaware of the pharmacist's legal position and may feel that the pharmacist is being judgmental and discriminative towards them. A consistent approach is required from all members of staff including locums. It will not help the situation if the patient is allowed to buy citric acid on one occasion and refused it on another.

Another area for consideration is that of display. Staff may find it easier to refuse a sale on the grounds that the item is not stocked at the pharmacy, as opposed to refusing a sale of an item that the patient can see. It would be beneficial, both from a harm minimisation point of view, and as a way of reducing the potential for conflict, for the patient to be directed to a non-pharmacy service which can respond to the request.

Over-the-counter medication
Not all drug misuse involves illicit drug use. Some people misuse prescribed medicines and others misuse OTCs. (Much of this is covered in Chapter 13.) It is advisable to check with your nearest drug agency and the local CD inspector, which OTC medication is commonly misused in the area. Consideration should then be given as to whether to display this medication or to keep it out of sight, to make it easier to refuse a sale. However, it is important to remember that drug users are not immune to colds, coughs, flu and headaches, constipation and disturbed sleep. More information on the healthcare of drug users can be found in Chapter 14.

MANAGING SOME OF THESE ISSUES
Many of the issues outlined above can be prevented if a number of measures are put into place before problems occur. Thinking ahead, and planning for the emergence of problems, is always better than "crisis management" when a problem actually occurs. First and foremost, however, is the importance of maintaining a positive non-judgmental approach to drug misuse and drug users. Building positive working relationships with patients and other service users will help to minimise the escalation of minor incidents into major catastrophes.

Ensuring procedures are efficient, effective, legal and understood by all involved
Communication between all the professionals involved in patient care is essential. Clinics and prescribing doctors should be aware of the pharmacy's opening hours and which services are provided. If the patient attends a specialist drug clinic, always find out who their drug worker is and get their contact number.

If at all possible, educate local prescribing doctors and drug workers to phone before they send a new patient. This provides time in which to decide whether you can take on any more patients, and hence avoids the embarrassment and offence of having to refuse a patient face-to-face. It also provides an opportunity to gain information on the patient, such as starting dose, what type of treatment they are receiving, and if there are any relevant medical or behavioural problems of which you should be aware. It also provides a chance to discuss "house rules" with the prescriber/drug worker, and procedures for feedback. This should also help when drawing up "Patient Agreements" at the start of treatment (see below).

One of the best ways to minimise problems is to ensure that services are as efficient as possible while maintaining a legal, ethical and professional stance. It may be a good idea to audit the service, and take a good look at how things are done, where they tend to go wrong and how such events can be minimised. For instance, problems are likely to occur when a new prescription for methadone is not at the pharmacy after the old one has run out. Routinely reminding patients a few days in advance to make sure they have a new prescription, or contacting the prescribing doctor or drug team to do the same, could minimise any problems. Ensure that all staff and locums are aware of the procedures.

Locums

Locums may be seen as a "soft touch" by patients as they are often not fully aware of "house rules". Therefore, locums need to be briefed about local agreements regarding service provision and may also need to be given training. In situations where the pharmacy normally provides services such as the supply of injecting equipment either by sale or through a needle exchange, or dispensing methadone prescriptions, the locum should be made aware of this. They should be talked through all of the procedures and other practical issues such as days when patients normally pick up their medication, what time they normally come in, and any potential problems. Where a pharmacist has made a decision not to provide services for whatever reason, the locum should not take it upon themselves to commence such services without discussing it with the regular pharmacist. A well-informed locum will be better equipped to avoid potential conflict situations. A useful publication for locums is published by the Pharmaceutical Press (Mason, 1998).

Building relationships with other members of the care team

Often cited as one of the main reasons pharmacists choose to opt out of providing services is the fact that they feel unsupported when providing services to drug users. This is of particular importance in the context of managing problems and incidents, when they may have experienced little or no support from GPs and other prescribers.

If the pharmacist has a good working relationship with other agencies, and where both parties understand the constraints under which each works, incidents can be either avoided or dealt with smoothly. For example, many drug workers or doctors may not consider the implications of an incorrectly written CD prescription or, as mentioned previously, may refer patients to pharmacies for ancillary injecting paraphernalia.

It is also advisable to discuss local and in-house "rules" with prescribing services, as it is important that everyone gives out the same message. This can be accomplished by providing these agencies with a list of the services offered by the pharmacy, during which times, and pharmacy contact details. You can also request similar information from them and build good communication links between all parties concerned.

Limit numbers if services are very much in demand

Because methadone patients tend to take up more time than other patients, as many come in daily, some pharmacists decide to limit the number of drug users to whom they feel they can provide a methadone dispensing service. Sometimes, when commencing service provision, pharmacists decide to take on only one or two patients, but when they see that service provision is a relatively simple and trouble-free process they agree to take on more.

As a general rule, providing this service should not interfere with or inhibit service provision to other patients, but if a pharmacy is in an area of high demand, it may come under pressure either from drug users, methadone prescribers or counselling services to take on more patients. At this point, a decision has to be taken as to whether it is practical and feasible to expand the service or to refer to another pharmacy in the area. As patient numbers grow, there will be a need to increase levels of security, staff awareness and training, as well as reviewing procedures.

Patient agreements – what both sides will do

As more doctors decide that their methadone patients should take their methadone under supervision at the pharmacy, many pharmacists will find themselves being part of a group of pharmacists asked to offer this service. In some localities, services have become formalised, with the health authority paying pharmacists and ensuring they have received adequate training. More about this type of service can be found in Chapter 17.

One useful tool, often employed when providing this service, is the use of the "patient agreement". This is a document which outlines what the pharmacist will provide in terms of service, and what is expected of the patient. Other elements included in the agreement may be details of when the pharmacist will withhold the dose, such as when the patient is intoxicated, what times to come in, coming to the pharmacy alone. In addition to the agreement, the pharmacist can also have "house rules" which could include the fact that shoplifting will never be tolerated and will result in the dispensing service, or needle exchange service, being withdrawn. The agreement can also deal with issues such as confidentiality, stating what information will be shared with whom.

Although normally associated with supervised methadone dispensing, there is no reason why such agreements cannot be devised, in consultation with local treatment services, for all methadone patients. Agreements can be written or verbal. An example of a written agreement for supervised methadone is provided in Figure 11.1.

While the document is not legally binding, it does provide a framework for discussions with patients about how the service will be operated and what sort of behaviour will not be tolerated. Essentially, use of such a document encourages pharmacists to talk to patients about these issues at the start of treatment and to discuss the ground rules in a positive, non-judgmental manner.

Security of premises

Maintaining a "drug habit" can be very expensive, and for some drug users, a major source of money is through engaging in illegal activities.

Pharmacists report that one of the many problems they face is methadone patients and needle exchange patients who shoplift, and this is undoubtedly an issue. However, it is often not the patient who shoplifts, but their associates, so asking patients to come into the pharmacy alone may help with this. If a patient is caught shoplifting, he/she can be banned from the pharmacy and, if appropriate, the prescribing doctor or drug team can be informed.

What the Client will do:
- *Drink the methadone in front of the pharmacist when required to do so*
- *Treat pharmacy staff with respect*
- *Attend the pharmacy daily within agreed times*
- *Not attend intoxicated with alcohol and/or drugs*
- *Attend alone and leave pets outside*
- *In exceptional circumstances, wait or return later if the pharmacist is busy*
- *Attend the "clinic" / GP for a reassessment if you have not attended the pharmacy for three days or more*
- *Not allow any other person to attend the pharmacy on your behalf unless previously arranged by the "clinic / GP"*
- *Be aware that the pharmacy may have to pass on necessary information about your case to the "clinic" / GP on a "need to know" basis*

What the pharmacist will do:
- *Provide a confidential/private space for your methadone supervision*
- *Keep records of your attendance*
- *Have responsibility for your care*
- *Dispense methadone in accordance with the prescription (for example, missed doses will not be supplied at a later date)*
- *Liaise when necessary with the "clinic" / GP with regard to your treatment*
- *Refer you back to the "clinic" / GP and NOT dispense your methadone if you do not attend the pharmacy for three days or more, as your tolerance to your methadone dose may have fallen. If you attend intoxicated your methadone will not be dispensed for that day. If your behaviour causes any problems, you will also be referred back to the "clinic" / GP*
- *NOT dispense your methadone to a representative unless previously authorised by the "clinic" / GP*
- *Provide health promotion and education*

Date:

Client: **Pharmacist:**
Name: **Name:**

Signature: **Signature:**

Figure 11.1 Supervised Administration of Methadone in the Community Pharmacy Client/ Pharmacist Agreement Form (adapted from Croydon supervised methadone scheme 1997).

Shoplifting is a potential problem with any patients or customers who use the pharmacy. Pharmacists and their staff need to feel confident that they are able to deal with this situation should it arise. Retail environments have "tempting tools of the trade" for the drug user such as cash, and in the case of pharmacy, drugs as well. Community pharmacies are generally open to the public, are open long hours and have their wares on display. Many pharmacies have decided to install CCTV and panic buttons (in several positions front and back of the shop). In some cases, these have been funded by local health authorities.

Fortunately, more serious events such as being held up by armed individuals for money and/or drugs are extremely rare events (Smith and Weidner, 1996a,b; Sheridan *et al*, 2000). Precautions can be taken to prevent such events occurring;

these include ensuring sufficient staffing levels at all times, appropriate training for staff and appropriate safety precautions in place e.g. panic buttons in accessible places. Everyone in the pharmacy should know when to use it, and not necessarily wait for the person in charge to do so, as they may be involved in dealing with the situation.

Security issues also extend to being broken into after hours, and the installation of adequate security measures is essential. Concerns need to extend beyond concerns with security of stock and premises. The security of staff and other customers is of paramount importance. All staff should feel confident that they can prevent, diffuse, and deal with violent or aggressive incidents.

MANAGING AND DIFFUSING VIOLENT INCIDENTS

The RPSGB recently convened a working party to look at the issue of service provision by community pharmacists to drug users. One of their key recommendations was that these services should be carried out in such a way that staff, customers and premises remain safe (RPSGB, 1998). There is no foolproof way of dealing with aggression, and there is no real substitute for "hands on" training. However, the following suggestions may well help to prevent or diffuse a situation. Pharmacists need to be organised in their working practices, have safe systems of working, and ground rules. They should make these clear to staff so that a consistent approach is followed. Inconsistencies can cause major problems.

A number of factors can be potential causes of such incidents. These include: patient inability to communicate effectively or to feel that one is understood, the use of illegal drugs or alcohol, protecting one's integrity, feeling threatened, misinterpreting information, group pressure, having been "rewarded" for violence in the past, authoritarian staff attitudes, fear and anxiety, being overwhelmed with information (Maudsley, 1994).

Pharmacy staff need to be able to recognise the signs of aggression early on. These include: increased agitation, pacing, flushed or pale complexion, raised tone of voice, clenched fists, banging of doors or furniture, and a tense atmosphere. Non-verbal signs of stress are often similar to those of anger and may be misinterpreted by pharmacists and staff, who may take such behaviour "personally". This may then cause pharmacists and staff to "mirror" this behaviour, which is likely to escalate the problem.

In the first instance one should try to verbally defuse a situation by calming down the situation, encouraging the patient to talk about the problem and showing that you understand their predicament and their point of view. Staff should try to have a calm and open posture, avoiding sudden movements, making appropriate eye contact and not standing facing the person, but moving to their side. Talking in a soft tone and taking things slowly will help to calm the situation and avoiding an audience is also a good idea. In trying to help the individual to solve the problem without resorting to violence, it is helpful to try and address the problem in small steps and to try and offer solutions or alternatives at each stage without the person having to "lose face".

It is essential not to try and manage situations alone – always call for help. The safety of staff and other customers is paramount. Situations which appear to be escalating out of control may require a call for back-up from other staff or from the police. In such circumstances, it is important to continue to talk to the person and to make it clear that the situation is unacceptable and ask him/her to leave. It is important also to be aware of your "exits", in case violence does occur.

What to do after an event has occurred

Violent and aggressive events are likely to leave staff feeling shocked or upset and angry, and staff may feel numbed for a couple of hours afterwards. As the effects of adrenaline wear off, many people begin to feel upset or tired, and it may be inappropriate for them to drive home. All those involved in an incident should be allowed to express their feelings preferably in a neutral environment with a neutral person. Talking about how they felt before, during and after the incident is important and individuals need to be allowed to express any anger they feel relating to the incident. Staff may need some time off work and should continue to receive support once they return.

Documenting the incident at the time is essential and this should include details of anyone who witnessed the event, encouraging them to document it independently. It may be some time before the issue is dealt with.

A decision will need to be made about whether or how to continue service provision for the individual involved. Decisions will be easier to make if other members of staff and the patients' care team are consulted. If the individual is a methadone patient, the prescribing doctor or drug team should be informed. However, remember – such incidents are rare and even rarer if the pharmacist is well-prepared, supported and has a positive attitude.

CONCLUSION

This chapter has focussed on problems and difficulties which may arise when providing services to drug users. However, it is essential to bear in mind the valuable contribution that the community pharmacist can make, and the relatively smooth conduct of these services. Finally, involvement in providing services for drug users can be a very rewarding part of a pharmacist's job, providing many opportunities for inter-professional collaboration, being part of a team approach to care and building positive professional relationships with patients.

REFERENCES

Departments of Health *et al.* (1999). *Drug Misuse and Dependence: Guidelines on Clinical Management*, The Stationery Office, London.
Mason PM (1998). *Locum Pharmacy*, Pharmaceutical Press, London.
Matheson C (1998). Privacy and stigma in the pharmacy: the illicit drug user's perspective and implications for pharmacy practice. *Pharmaceutical Journal*, 260, 639–641.
Matheson C, Bond CM, Mollison J (1999). Attitudinal factors associated with community pharmacists' involvement in services for drug misusers. *Addiction*, 94, 1349–1359.
Maudsley Hospital (1994). *Preventing and Managing Violence. Policy and Guidelines for Practice. Report of the Trust Working Party.* Maudsley Hospital, London.
RPSGB (1998). *Report of Working Party on Pharmaceutical Services for Drug Misusers: A Report to the Council of the Royal Pharmaceutical Society of Great Britain*, RPSGB, London.
Sheridan J, Strang J, Barber, N, Glanz A (1996). Role of community pharmacies in relation to HIV prevention and drug misuse: findings from the 1995 national survey in England and Wales. *British Medical Journal*, 313, 272–274.

Sheridan J, Strang J, Taylor C, Barber N (1997). HIV prevention and drug treatment services for drug misusers: a national study of community pharmacists' attitudes and their involvement in service specific training. *Addiction*, 92, 1737–1748.

Sheridan J, Lovell S, Turnbull P, Parsons J, Stimson G, Strang J (2000). Pharmacy-based needle exchange (PBNX) schemes in south-east England: Survey of service providers. *Addiction*, 95, 1551–1560.

Smith F, Weidner D (1996a). Threatening and violent incidents in community pharmacies. Part 1: An investigation of the frequency of serious and minor incidents. *International Journal of Pharmacy Practice*, 4, 136–144.

Smith F, Weidner D (1996b). Threatening and violent incidents in community pharmacies. Part 2: Implications for pharmacists and community pharmacy services. *International Journal of Pharmacy Practice*, 4, 145–152.

12

New approaches to dispensing controlled drugs: supervised consumption of methadone

Laurence Gruer and Kay Roberts

INTRODUCTION

Methadone has become established as the standard medical treatment for opiate dependence in many countries. In most of these countries, it can only be prescribed by a doctor if it is taken by the patient under the direct supervision of a professional, typically in a specialist clinic (Farrell *et al.*, 1994; Harkin *et al.*, 1997; Ward *et al.*, 1999). The United Kingdom is unusual in that doctors can prescribe methadone in any dosage form and not necessarily for dispensing in daily instalments. This means that patients can present a prescription for methadone at a community pharmacy and leave the shop with a large quantity of methadone in the form of oral mixture, tablets or ampoules for use as they see fit. Recently, there has been growing recognition in the United Kingdom that this has led to widespread misuse and diversion of methadone onto the illicit market, diminishing the effectiveness of treatment and contributing to a growing number of methadone-related deaths (Cairns *et al.*, 1996).

In 1999, revised guidelines on the clinical management of drug misuse and dependence were issued by the United Kingdom Departments of Health (Departments of Health, 1999). These now explicitly recommend that new patients should consume methadone under supervision, for the first few months at least. This important policy shift has major implications for community pharmacists in the United Kingdom who will often be the professionals best placed to provide the supervision.

In this chapter, we first consider the rationale for supervising the consumption of methadone. We then examine how one area, Greater Glasgow, has successfully developed a system enabling around 3,000 patients to consume their daily methadone under the supervision of community pharmacists. The mechanics of the system are described and its benefits considered. How various practical problems can be overcome is discussed.

WHY SUPERVISED CONSUMPTION CAN HELP

There are three main reasons why supervising the consumption of controlled drugs prescribed in the treatment of drug dependence makes sense. First, it can ensure that the treatment is taken in the dose and at the time prescribed, by the person for whom it was intended – i.e. it improves compliance and the likelihood of health benefit from treatment. Secondly, it can prevent diversion onto the black market and misuse by others thereby reducing risks of inadvertent overdose by the opiate naïve user, for example. And finally, it can prevent deaths resulting from accidental ingestion of prescribed methadone by children (Beattie, 1999).

Supervised consumption would be unnecessary if drug dependent patients could be relied upon to take their treatment as prescribed. However, there are a number of reasons why they often do not or cannot comply with this regimen. In some cases, they may wish to vary the dose in order to alter the psychoactive effect of the drug. They may also see the prescribed drug as second-rate, to be replaced if possible by their "drug of choice", for which they may part-exchange or sell their prescribed drug. Without supervision, the doctor has little or no control over what happens to the prescription and the dispensing pharmacist must simply watch the drugs disappear out the pharmacy door to an unknown fate.

The extent of diversion of prescribed controlled drugs can be illustrated by reports on the drugs used by new attenders at drug misuse services in Scotland in the year up to April 1998. Table 12.1 shows that among individuals reporting use of methadone, dihydrocodeine and diazepam, 38%, 64% and 68% respectively had not obtained them on prescription. In the case of temazepam, almost 90% had not been prescribed to the user. These data demonstrate both the propensity of drug misusers to use pharmaceutical drugs and their ready availability on the black market. While the exact source of pharmaceutical drugs on the black market is usually unknown, it is clear that a substantial proportion derives from diverted individual prescriptions.

THE CASE FOR SUPERVISING THE CONSUMPTION OF METHADONE
Numerous studies world-wide have shown that when properly used, oral methadone mixture is a highly effective substitute for heroin, achieving large reductions in the frequency of injecting, illicit opiate use, incidence of overdose and death, and drug-related crime (Farrell *et al.*, 1994; Ward *et al.*, 1999). However, such studies have mainly been conducted in the USA and involved patients most of whom were receiving methadone under supervision. On the other hand, until very recently, nearly all the methadone prescribed in the United Kingdom was dispensed for consumption without supervision (Strang *et al.*, 1996). We do not know how much of this methadone was actually taken by the individuals to whom it was prescribed. But we do know, as Table 12.1 shows,

Table 12.1 Pharmaceutical drugs misused by new attenders at drug misuse services in Scotland in year ending 31 March 1998

	All reports	Prescribed	Non-prescribed	% Non-prescribed
Methadone	2489	1539	950	38
Dihydrocodeine	3413	1228	2185	64
Diazepam	1709	1541	1168	68
Temazepam	1104	158	946	86

Source: *Drug Misuse Statistics Scotland, 1998 Bulletin.* ISD Scotland, Edinburgh 1999.

that the misuse of non-prescribed methadone has been common in Scotland. In addition, methadone also now makes a substantial contribution to drug-related deaths in England and Wales. The St George's national programme on drug-related deaths recorded 703 deaths in the first six months of 1999, including 40 (6%) where methadone was the only substance implicated and 104 (18%) where methadone was implicated with other drugs (Ghodse *et al.*, 2000). In 56 of the 144 cases the methadone had not been prescribed to the deceased. There is thus good reason to believe that the practice of dispensing prescribed methadone for consumption without supervision in the United Kingdom provides almost limitless opportunities for its misuse, thereby reducing benefits to patients and increasing risks to patients and others.

As the professional responsible for dispensing most of the methadone mixture prescribed in the United Kingdom, the community pharmacist is ideally placed to supervise its consumption, thereby contributing importantly to the treatment of patients and the protection of the wider community. However, supervised dispensing is not at present part of the community pharmacist's contract: pharmacists can choose whether or not to offer this service. How, then, can pharmacists take on such a role? What are the requirements? What are the pitfalls? A high level of involvement by pharmacists in the supervision of methadone began in Greater Glasgow in 1994. The rest of this chapter describes how these arrangements came about, how they have worked in practice and what lessons can be learned from the experience.

A BRIEF HISTORY OF METHADONE PRESCRIBING IN GLASGOW

During the 1970s and until 1981, methadone was only prescribed by psychiatrists specialising in addiction in Glasgow to a small group of heroin dependent patients. In 1981, there was a rapid increase in heroin injecting in the city's council estates and the number of patients attending the drug misuse clinics soared (Ditton and Speirits, 1982). Without adequate support and monitoring facilities, the service was overwhelmed and methadone prescribing was abandoned in favour of a drug-free approach (Drummond *et al.*, 1986). Without any specialist support for methadone prescribing, many of the city's GPs began prescribing other opiates such as dihydrocodeine and buprenorphine tablets, in the hope of reducing their patients' reliance on injected heroin. By the end of the decade, buprenorphine had become the most popular injected drug in Glasgow and dihydrocodeine tablets were also widely available for sale on the streets. In the absence of any coherent policy, prescribing anarchy reigned.

In the late 1980s, physicians at the city's infectious diseases unit began prescribing oral methadone to their drug injecting patients who were infected with HIV, in an attempt to stabilise their health and reduce the risk of HIV transmission to others through needle sharing (Greater Glasgow Health Board, 1992). Consumption of the methadone was unsupervised. In 1991, a small number of general practitioners began to use methadone in a more systematic way with their own patients, receiving help in counselling and non-medical support from local drug agencies. Keen to ensure that their patients took the methadone as prescribed, especially when a relatively high dose was required, they made informal arrangements with local community pharmacists to observe patients swallowing their methadone in the pharmacy. They found that in most cases, these arrangements worked extremely well, often resulting in dramatic improvements in their patients' health and well-being (Wilson *et al.*, 1994).

In 1993, Greater Glasgow Health Board agreed a revised drug misuse strategy (Gruer, 1993). Key objectives included reducing the prevalence of injecting, reducing the number of drug-related deaths and holding the prevalence of HIV among injectors to below 1.5%. The strategy likened the required services to a series of stepping stones, each one enabling drug injectors to progress as far from harmful drug use as they could at the time. The main suggested steps were: needle exchanges to reduce equipment sharing; methadone programmes to reduce injecting; and detoxification and rehabilitation programmes to reduce drug dependency and to come off drugs altogether. Based on the available evidence, methadone was identified as the medical intervention with the greatest potential for reducing morbidity and mortality. Given the extent of drug injecting in the city and the favourable experience of the pioneering GPs, general practice was seen as the preferred setting for most methadone prescribing to be carried out. However, it was recognised that, in order to succeed, GPs needed support from medical specialists, drug counsellors and community pharmacists.

The model for the specialist medical service was the Community Drug Problem Service (CDPS) in Edinburgh, established in 1988 (Greenwood, 1990); this service took referrals of opiate injectors from general practitioners and others, assessed the patient, initiated treatment with methadone where appropriate and then returned the patient to his or her GP for ongoing care. With this approach, the CDPS had achieved remarkable success in encouraging a high proportion of GPs in Edinburgh to treat patients with methadone, leading to a large reduction in the proportion of opiate addicts in Edinburgh who were injecting. However, the methadone was prescribed for dispensing without supervision.

When it opened in January 1994, the Glasgow Drug Problem Service (GDPS) differed in two main ways from its Edinburgh equivalent. Firstly, all patients could only be referred by their GP who also had to agree in advance to continue prescribing methadone if this was successfully initiated by the GDPS. This was to prevent patients accumulating at the GDPS and to increase the number of GPs involved in the prescribing of methadone. In addition to this, the GDPS aimed to arrange with community pharmacists for all patients to take their methadone under supervision. It was felt that, unless a secure system for administering methadone was established from the outset, the effectiveness of the service would be compromised and it would not obtain the support of either GPs or the general public.

A survey, undertaken by the Area Pharmaceutical Committee (APC) and the GDPS in early 1994, found that 46% of the city's 210 community pharmacists were dispensing methadone and 20% were already voluntarily supervising consumption (Scott *et al.*, 1994). Following this favourable response, the APC recommended that supervised consumption of methadone should become standard practice within the Glasgow area, although pharmacists' involvement should remain entirely voluntary.

Also in 1994, the Health Board established the GP Drug Misuse Clinic Scheme (Gruer *et al.*, 1997). This followed lengthy negotiations between the Health Board and the Local Medical Committee representing general practitioners. The Health Board accepted the principle that GPs who treated drug dependent patients in a systematic and ongoing way merited extra payment for the additional work involved. It was agreed that, to be eligible for additional payments, GPs had to have a minimum of five opiate dependent patients; to follow written guidelines on assessment and treatment;

to arrange for additional counselling and support from a drug counsellor or trained nurse; to attend at least two training seminars a year; and to submit data regularly. In addition, "daily methadone self-administration under the supervision of a nominated community pharmacist should be arranged whenever possible". At the outset, 39 GPs joined the scheme. By 1996, the number had grown to 75 and by 2001 to 168, representing over 40% of all practices in the Health Board area.

FORMALISING ARRANGEMENTS WITH COMMUNITY PHARMACISTS
With the establishment of the GDPS and the GP Clinic Scheme, the annual number of daily methadone doses supervised by community pharmacists rose from a few thousand in 1993 to over 180,000 in the 12 months after the new services began in April 1994. Consequently, the additional workload for many community pharmacists became considerable. In March 1995 the Health Board decided to pay an additional fee to pharmacists who agreed to supervise the self-administration of methadone on their premises to a written standard. Fees were banded to reflect the number of supervisions undertaken per month and the number of days per week that the pharmacy was open. In order to encourage as much daily supervision as possible, the highest fees were paid to those pharmacies supervising consumption seven days a week for a high number of patients. Contracting pharmacies are required to keep a log of the number of supervised and unsupervised doses of methadone dispensed each day and to submit this quarterly.

By April 1996, 125 (59%) of the community pharmacies in the Health Board area had contracted to provide a supervision service, and by mid-2000 had risen to 167 (78%). During the first four years of these arrangements, the number of supervisions continued to rise, exceeding 600,000 in 1998/99 (see Figure 12.1). By 2001, an estimated 3,000 patients were receiving supervised methadone each day, representing about 80% of all patients receiving methadone in Glasgow. This equates to an average of around 18 patients per participating pharmacy. However, patients being prescribed methadone are not evenly distributed throughout the area, but live largely

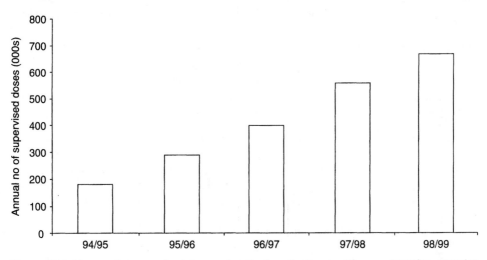

Figure 12.1 Pharmacist-supervised doses of methadone in Greater Glasgow 1994/95–1998/99.

in areas of socio-economic deprivation. In addition, pharmacies differ in the number of patients they can handle. Consequently, the number of patients supervised at each pharmacy varies enormously from two or three to around 100. Around 80% of the participating pharmacies provide the service six days weekly and 12% seven days weekly. Most of the remaining pharmacies (dispensing five days weekly) are situated in health centres, which are not open at the weekend.

SUPERVISION IN PRACTICE

The practical, legal and ethical implications of supervising the consumption of methadone are also covered in Chapters 9 and 11. Guidelines have been produced for pharmacists who have contracted to provide supervision. These are jointly published by the Greater Glasgow Area Pharmaceutical Committee, Health Board and Primary Care Trust (2000). They include information on the payment structure of the scheme as well as practical guidance on managing the supervised consumption of methadone in the community pharmacy. Issues such as privacy, confidentiality, missed doses, behaviour of clients in the pharmacy and communication with prescribers are covered in detail.

All pharmacy staff involved, including locum pharmacists, need to understand the procedures involved in providing the service. Each pharmacy should thus have its own written protocol to ensure continuity of service and reduce the chance of problems arising. This should cover dealing with new and regular patients, preparation of doses, supervision procedure, missed doses, intoxicated patients and record keeping. It is recommended that the pharmacist ensures that patients have swallowed the methadone by asking them to wash the dose down with a small drink of water and engage in conversation to ensure their mouth is emptied.

Patient contracts or agreements are highly recommended and most participating pharmacists in Glasgow now have these. They may be either verbal or written and should address behaviour in the pharmacy, collection times, missed doses and intoxication. Patients should be made aware from the outset that missed doses cannot be replaced. Intoxicated patients are advised of the danger of overdose and that their dose will be withheld and they may be asked to return to consume their dose later that day.

SUPPORT AND TRAINING FOR COMMUNITY PHARMACISTS SINCE 1995

To support community pharmacists involved in dispensing methadone, providing needle exchange, and other work with drug misusers, the Health Board created a new post of Area Pharmacy Specialist – Drug Misuse in 1996. The responsibilities of this post included the following:

1. To function as an advocate for the supervised self-administration of methadone;
2. To provide support and advice to pharmacists involved in the continuing care of drug misusers;
3. To monitor and evaluate the supervised consumption of methadone;
4. To co-ordinate and monitor the free pharmacy needle and syringe exchange service within the overall programme;
5. To provide pharmaceutical input into the strategic development of local services for drug misusers.

It was recognised that pharmacists involved in dispensing and supervising methadone would require additional training if they were fully to develop this role. Continuing education for all pharmacists in Scotland is provided from the Scottish Centre for Post-qualification Pharmaceutical Education (SCPPE) based at the University of Strathclyde. In conjunction with practising pharmacists in Glasgow, SCPPE developed a distance-learning package on methadone (Mackie, 1996). This gives an overview of the rationale for the use of methadone in the treatment of opiate dependence. Its completion has now become a requirement for Glasgow pharmacists entering the contracted supervision programme. A more comprehensive package examining the wider role of the community pharmacist in the care of the drug misuser has also been developed for pharmacists providing free needle exchange and is available as an additional option (Parr and Brailey, 1999). Joint continuing education meetings are held at least annually at which GPs and pharmacists involved in methadone prescribing and dispensing can discuss matters of common interest. In addition to the above, pharmacists are encouraged to complete an accredited health promotion training programme and another SCPPE distant-learning package "Scotland's Health: Challenge for a Pharmacy", both of which include sections on health promotion aspects of drug misuse and sexual health. SCPPE educational events in Glasgow have included drug misuse and the treatment of opiate dependence, misuse of over-the-counter medicines, the nutritional status of drug misusers, their dental and oral health and hepatitis C.

Supervising the consumption of methadone raises a number of issues for community pharmacists. Some of the commonest and how they have been tackled are discussed below:

Numbers

Swallowing an average dose of 50–60 ml of methadone mixture does not usually take long. However, the pharmacist will inevitably spend more time supervising the patient and completing any additional paperwork than if the methadone had simply been dispensed as a take-home dose. Large numbers of patients requiring supervision can thus place considerable strain on staff and be unpopular with other customers. Pharmacists have adopted a variety of approaches to minimise the impact on other customers. Most have decided upon the maximum number of supervised patients they can reasonably manage. Some arrange for patients to come during otherwise quiet periods of the day, while others try to spread supervised patients more evenly through the day.

Privacy

Some supervised patients have expressed a dislike of having to swallow their methadone in full view of other customers, thereby drawing attention to the fact that they are drug addicts. Their presence in the pharmacy may be regarded with suspicion and concern by some customers. In order to increase the level of privacy, a growing number of pharmacies in Glasgow have created private areas where the patient is partly or wholly screened from other customers. These can be used not only for patients receiving methadone, but also for needle and syringe exchange or discreet discussion with any customer on a wide range of issues. Greater Glasgow

Health Board and Drug Action Team have made specific funding available for this purpose.

Communication with GPs
The Greater Glasgow GP Drug Misuse Clinic Scheme Guidelines (Greater Glasgow Health Board, 1999) urge prescribing doctors to agree with the patient from which pharmacy they wish to receive their methadone. The GP should then contact the preferred pharmacy to establish whether they can take on a new patient and, if so, to provide the patient's name. To facilitate this, doctors in the scheme can consult the pharmaceutical list which indicates those pharmacies providing supervision, classified by postcode. However, some GPs still do not contact the pharmacist and patients may simply arrive at the pharmacy with a prescription upon which the doctor has requested supervision. Efforts are being made to emphasise to all participating GPs the importance of direct communication with the dispensing pharmacist. GPs and pharmacists are also strongly encouraged to communicate with each other about sudden deterioration in the patient's condition or other problems such as missed doses, intoxicated patients or bad behaviour in and around the pharmacy.

Needle exchange for the patient on methadone
Some of the pharmacies providing supervision also offer a free needle and syringe exchange service and from time to time, patients receiving methadone will ask for needles and syringes, indicating that they are still injecting. This can create a dilemma for the pharmacist, aware that the use of methadone should ideally lead to the cessation of injecting. However, the pharmacist may have the opportunity to discuss with the patient the reasons for continued injecting, for example, because too low a dose of methadone is being prescribed. With the patient's agreement, this can lead to a dialogue between the pharmacist and the prescribing doctor or specialist service. Without the patient's consent, it is however crucial that confidentiality is maintained. Pharmacists providing needle exchange have been advised that it is essential that any injector is given a supply of clean injecting equipment.

Shoplifting
A large proportion of drug misusers raise money for buying drugs through shoplifting – a skill at which they can become expert. Although the evidence is clear that patients on methadone commit far fewer offences than untreated addicts (Hutchinson *et al.*, 2000), the risk still remains. Losses can, however, be minimised by making it clear to patients at the outset that shoplifting will be reported to both the police and the prescribing doctor and that the pharmacist can and will refuse to dispense the methadone. Allowing only one patient into the shop at a time and discouraging accompanying friends can also reduce the risk. In practice, few of the participating pharmacists have found this to be major problem.

HOW LONG SHOULD SUPERVISION BE CONTINUED?
The decision to reduce or discontinue supervision rests with the prescribing doctor. At present, there are a wide variety of views on when this should happen. The latest

Table 12.2 Proportion of respondents (n = 90) indicating each criterion for relaxing the supervised consumption of methadone

Criterion	% respondents
Employment responsibilities	39
Very low dose/low dose	35
Good compliance/stable/trustworthy	31
Good evidence of no misuse/clean urine	16
Travel/holidays	12
Personal circumstances/good reason	6
Illness	6
Parental/relative/domestic supervision	6
Longer than one year in treatment	2
Reducing/coming off/trying to come off	2
Gut impression	1

United Kingdom "Clinical guidelines on the management of drug misuse" (Departments of Health, 1999) suggest supervision should continue for a minimum of three months. An authoritative report on reducing drug-related deaths recommends six months (Advisory Council on the Misuse of Drugs, 2000). In Greater Glasgow, it has been found that this is usually too short and a minimum of twelve months is advised (Greater Glasgow Health Board, 1999). It is clear however that relaxing supervision can be an important step in the patient's rehabilitation. The crucial question is whether or not the patient can be relied upon to take his or her methadone responsibly without supervision. In a recent survey of GPs in the Glasgow scheme, a wide range of reasons for reducing supervision were given (Table 12.2). A sensible approach is to reduce supervision gradually with a continued requirement for daily dispensing with supervision every second day at the outset, moving to once a week if progress is satisfactory. In this respect, the pharmacist's involvement can be helpful, both in guiding the prescriber as to whether less supervision would be sensible and in alerting him to any problems thereafter.

DOES SUPERVISION WORK?

The huge proportion of pharmacists joining the Glasgow scheme reflects the widely held view that supervising the consumption of methadone does make sense professionally, thus increasing pharmacists' confidence that this potentially dangerous drug will be used as intended by the prescriber. At the individual level, most participating pharmacists have found that the daily contact with patients on methadone enables them to get to know their patients much better and recognise changes in their health and circumstances. In most cases, pharmacists find that treatment with methadone results in striking improvements in the patient's health and well-being.

A follow-up study of patients receiving methadone in Glasgow has shown marked improvements at six and twelve months compared with their pre-treatment state (Hutchinson *et al.*, 2000). Benefits included large reductions in the frequency

Table 12.3 Methadone-related deaths and quantity of methadone prescribed in Greater Glasgow and Lothian, Scotland in 1996 and 1997

	All drug-related deaths	Methadone-related deaths	Quantity of methadone prescribed	Deaths per kg of methadone
Greater Glasgow	165	41	92.2	0.44
Lothian	99	66	46.4	1.42

Source: *Drug Misuse Statistics Scotland, 1997 and 1998 Bulletins.* ISD Scotland, 1998, 1999.

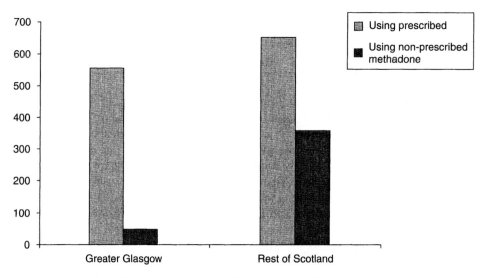

Source: *Drug Misuse Statistics Scotland, 1998 Bulletin.* ISD Scotland

Figure 12.2 New attenders at drug misuse services reporting main drug as prescribed or non-prescribed methadone.

of injecting and injecting-related health problems, illicit opiate use and drug-related crime and were most marked for those who remained continuously on treatment with methadone throughout the year of follow-up. In 1996 and 1997, less than half as much methadone was prescribed in the Edinburgh area (Lothian) – where there was little supervision – than in Greater Glasgow, but 61% more methadone-related deaths were recorded (Information and Statistics Division Scotland, 1998, 1999) (Table 12.3).

Scottish national figures from drug misuse services show that the proportion of new attenders reporting use of non-prescribed methadone is much lower in Greater Glasgow than in other parts of Scotland (Information and Statistics Division Scotland, 1999) (Figure 12.2). Consequently, there is good evidence that supervised

Table 12.4 The cost of treatment with methadone in Greater Glasgow 1998–99

	Attendances (000s)	Cost (£000s)	% total cost
Methadone mixture	–	810	26
Pharmacy dispensing fees	833	1623	53
Pharmacy supervision fees	661	393	13
GP scheme fees	46	256	8
Total		3082	100

consumption is helping both to prevent deaths and reduce the amount of methadone misuse. The additional cost of supervision depends upon the level of any fees paid and the proportion of methadone that is supervised. In Greater Glasgow, in 1998–99, supervision accounted for 13% of the total cost of the methadone programme (Table 12.4). The evidence suggests that this relatively modest increase in costs is being handsomely repaid in the improved health and behaviour of patients and the reductions in methadone diversion and methadone-related deaths.

CONCLUSION

It is increasingly accepted in the United Kingdom that supervised consumption is a crucial component of methadone prescribing (Departments of Health, 1999; Advisory Council on the Misuse of Drugs, 2000). The experience in Glasgow has shown that, by formalising arrangements for prescribing and supervising, large numbers of general practitioners and community pharmacists can become involved. This enables many more patients to be treated safely, to the benefit of both themselves and the wider community. With the apparently continuing increase in drug injecting across the country, it is clear that the role of the community pharmacist in this area will become ever more important. Adequate resourcing, training and support will be crucial if they are properly to fulfil this role. Given the success with methadone, the practicalities of supervising the self-administration of other potentially hazardous medications such as buprenorphine or benzodiazepines in the treatment of drug dependence should at least be explored.

REFERENCES

Advisory Council on the Misuse of Drugs (2000). *Reducing drug-related deaths*, Home Office, London.

Beattie J (1999). Children poisoned with illegal drugs in Glasgow. *British Medical Journal*, 318, 1137.

Cairns A, Roberts I, Benbow B (1996). Characteristics of fatal methadone overdose in Manchester, 1985–94. *British Medical Journal*, 313, 264–265.

Departments of Health (1999). *Drug misuse and dependence – Guidelines on Clinical Management*, The Stationery Office, London.

Ditton J, Speirits K (1982). The new wave of heroin addiction in Britain, *Sociology*, 16, 595–598.

Drummond CD, Taylor JA, Mullin PJ (1986). Replacement of a prescribing service by an opiate-free day programme in a Glasgow drug clinic. *British Journal of Addiction*, 81, 559–565.

Farrell M, Ward J, Mattick R, Hall W, Stimson G, des Jarlais D, *et al.*, (1994). Methadone maintenance treatment in opiate dependence: a review. *British Medical Journal*, 309, 997–1001.

Ghodse H, Oyefeso A, Lind J, Pollard M, Hunt M, Corkery J (2000). *Drug-related Deaths as reported by Coroners in England and Wales, January–June 1999*, St George's Hospital Medical School, London.

Greater Glasgow Area Pharmaceutical Committee, Greater Glasgow Health Board, Greater Glasgow Primary Care Trust (2000). *Guidelines for supervision of methadone consumption: Third edition* Glasgow.

Greater Glasgow Health Board (1992). *AIDS Control Act Report 1991–92*. GGHB, Glasgow.

Greater Glasgow Health Board (1999). *Guidelines for the Greater Glasgow GP Drug Misuse Clinic Scheme: Second edition* GGHB, Glasgow.

Greenwood J (1990). Creating a new drug service in Edinburgh. *British Medical Journal*, 300, 587–589.

Gruer L (1993). *Drug Misuse and Health in Greater Glasgow*, Greater Glasgow Health Board, Glasgow.

Gruer L, Wilson P, Scott R, Elliott L *et al.* (1997). General practitioner centred scheme for treatment of opiate dependent drug injectors in Glasgow. *British Medical Journal*, 414, 1730–1735.

Harkin A, Anderson P, Goos C (1997). *Smoking, drinking and drug taking in the European Region*. WHO Regional Office for Europe, Copenhagen.

Hutchinson S, Taylor A, Gruer L, Barr C, *et al.* (2000). One-year follow-up of opiate injectors treated with oral methadone in a GP-centred programme. *Addiction*, 95, 1055–1068.

ISD Scotland (1998). *Drug Misuse Statistics Scotland 1997*. Information and Statistics Division, Edinburgh.

ISD Scotland (1999). *Drug Misuse Statistics Scotland 1998*. Information and Statistics Division Scotland, Edinburgh.

Mackie C (1996). *Pharmaceutical aspects of methadone prescribing*, Scottish Centre for Post-qualification Pharmaceutical Education, Glasgow.

Parr R, Bailey A eds (1999). *Pharmaceutical care of the drug misuser*, Scottish Centre for Post-qualification Pharmaceutical Education, Glasgow.

Scott R, Burnett S, McNulty H (1994). Supervised administration of methadone by pharmacies. *British Medical Journal*, 308, 1438.

Strang J, Sheridan J, Barber N (1996). Prescribing injectable and oral methadone to opiate addicts: results from the 1995 national postal survey of community pharmacies in England and Wales. *British Medical Journal*, 313, 270–272.

Ward J, Hall W, Mattick R (1999). Role of maintenance treatment in opioid dependence. *Lancet*, 353, 221–226.

Wilson P, Watson R, Ralston G (1994). Methadone maintenance in general practice: patients, workload and outcomes. *British Medical Journal*, 309, 641–644.

13

Misuse of over-the-counter medicines in the UK: the prevention and management role for community pharmacists

David J Temple

INTRODUCTION

The cornerstone for the practice of all members of the pharmacy profession is "a prime concern for the welfare of the patient and other members of public"(RPSGB, 1999). Hence pharmacists have always considered themselves to be the guardians of the people with regard to drugs. As such they have been concerned about the inappropriate use of medicines which are sold "over the counter" (OTC) in their pharmacies. Indeed this concern is one of the main original arguments put forward to restrict medicine sales to pharmacies, rather than allow further products to become "General Sales List" and hence be available through any retail outlet such as supermarkets and garages.

Inappropriate use of OTCs includes patients with genuine minor illness, who are using a poor choice of preparation or an incorrect dosing of an effective remedy. In some cases, the patient continues to use the medication long after the condition has resolved. At the other extreme, some people may have deliberately experimented with OTC products to induce pleasurable effects or to mimic the effect produced by illicit drugs. Optimising the use of OTC drugs is outside the scope of this book and is best dealt with by education of the patient, through discussion in the pharmacy. The Royal Pharmaceutical Society of Great Britain (RPSGB) has been addressing this issue through the training of counter staff in effective questioning of customers, when making sales of OTC medicines. This chapter will consider primarily the "abuse" of OTC medicines, but will include a consideration of some products, where long term inappropriate use leads to problems of dependence.

WHO MISUSES OTCs?

Three types of people can be identified who are misusing these products.

a) persons who have used them legitimately for therapeutic reasons, but have used them excessively (high doses and/or for prolonged time periods) and have become physically or psychologically dependent to one or more of the constituents.

b)   persons who are deliberately experimenting with OTC products for non-medicinal purposes.
c)   persons who are dependent on harder drugs, but use OTC preparations as a substitute when other drugs are unavailable.

RESEARCH INTO THE MISUSE OF OTCs

Some limited research has been conducted on measuring the type and extent of misuse of OTC drugs. Most information is largely anecdotal, but many pharmacists will doubtless recognise all three groups amongst their customers. Ball and Wilde (1989) surveyed community pharmacists in West Cumbria by telephone and asked the question "do you have a problem with non-prescribed products being misused"? Twenty-four out of 25 pharmacists responded positively and identified codeine linctus as by far the most common suspect product. This was followed by kaolin and morphine mixture, laxatives and two former proprietary cough remedies containing antihistamines. In all, 21 products suspected of being misused were identified in this small study.

A more comprehensive postal survey was carried out by Paxton and Chapple (1996) in the neighbouring county in Northern England, Northumberland. Similar products were again identified by the pharmacists. Most reported at least one attempt to purchase a product for possible misuse during the previous month and had a policy for counter staff to refer the matter to the pharmacist. Specific strategies for dealing with clients were given, including not displaying such products and attempting to persuade clients to purchase an alternative product. Some pharmacists operated an impromptu grapevine with neighbouring pharmacies, although no formal schemes were in operation.

More recently, all Northern Ireland community pharmacies have been surveyed on their perceptions of the extent of OTC drug abuse, the drugs involved, the type of customers whom they suspect of abusing medicines, together with the methods they have used to deal with the problem (Hughes *et al.*, 1999). The 253 respondents (almost 50%) between them named 112 OTC products they perceived were being abused, and once again, opioids, antihistamines and laxatives topped the poll. Similar prevention strategies to the Northumberland pharmacists were also apparent. However, none of these studies has attempted to address this issue from the user's viewpoint.

PRODUCT TYPES MISUSED

Almost any substance can be misused (Wills, 1993). However, as reported above, of major concern are those agents that have a direct action on the central nervous system and cause a stimulant or depressant effect on mood. This includes pain-killers, anti-diarrhoeals, cough and cold preparations, travel sickness tablets and hay fever preparations. Pharmacologically, three main groups of drugs can be distinguished: opiate-like drugs, sedative drugs (such as the anti-histamines) and stimulant drugs (such as the sympathomimetics, which are structurally related to amphetamine). Many of these latter substances have been banned by the sporting authorities as potentially performance-enhancing. Two other groups of products are also of concern, namely volatile solvents which are most frequently misused by adolescents, and laxatives, the abuse of which has been mainly restricted to females.

The following sections will look briefly at specific drugs and other products which are liable to be misused.

Opioids

The main products here are codeine linctus and kaolin and morphine mixture. Although the latter may be used for its anti-diarrhoeal properties, there have been stories of heroin addicts decanting off the brown supernatant fluid and injecting it. The main side effects of OTC preparations are predicable from their pharmacological properties, such that codeine causes constipation. Other effects are less predicable, such as severe hypokalaemia resulting from prolonged use of kaolin and morphine mixture probably due to adsorption of potassium onto the kaolin in the gut.

Various other admixtures of opioids have achieved notoriety in the past, but their use is much more restricted nowadays as pharmacists have become aware of the abuse potential. These include J. Collis Browne's Mixture®, formerly Collis Browne's Chlorodyne®, which is still available as a pharmacy-only OTC product containing 1 mg anhydrous morphine in 5 ml. Likewise, Gee's Linctus (Opiate Squill Linctus, B.P. 1988) contains camphorated opium tincture. Most of the branded cough mixtures included a formulation "with codeine". However, these have also largely fallen by the wayside through increasing pharmacy vigilance as well as reformulation by the manufacturers.

Perhaps concern now should be centred on painkillers containing codeine with paracetamol (e.g. the heavily advertised Solpadeine®) and Paramol®, which contains dihydrocodeine with paracetamol. Solpadeine® also contains caffeine, which may increase its abuse potential. This and other issues relating to analgesic admixtures are covered in a subsequent section.

Antihistamines

Cyclizine poses a special problem. In the UK this antihistamine is still available for dispensing as Valoid® for the treatment of nausea, vomiting, vertigo, motion sickness and labyrinthine disorders. It is primarily used to prevent or treat vomiting during therapy with narcotic analgesics. In high doses it can cause euphoria and hallucinations, possibly due to its antimuscarinic properties. Diconal®, which contains dipipanone and cyclizine, was widely misused in some districts due to poor prescribing, until the Home Office required prescribers to obtain a licence to prescribe Diconal, since when prescribing has almost disappeared. However, knowledge of the effects of cyclizine may have caused some misusers with severe dependency to experiment with injecting cyclizine with methadone. The RPSGB has drawn pharmacists' attention to this problem and the code of ethics now instructs that cyclizine specifically should only be sold personally by the pharmacist (RPSGB, 1999). The fact that there is no suitable retail pack available now makes OTC sales very complicated anyway. Other antihistamines do not appear to have quite the same popularity with narcotic drug users. However, a separate group of mainly young users appears to exploit the interaction between the antihistamines and alcohol. In this case, liquid cough and cold preparations seem to be used, and pharmacists are usually on the alert when asked for such preparations by youngsters. Most of the older antihistamines cause drowsiness, an effect which is markedly increased when consumed together with alcohol.

Before leaving antihistamines, it is worth recalling a specific incident which occurred in 1997, which illustrates again the ingenuity of determined drug users. In that year, a product called Sleepia® (diphenhydramine) was introduced into the British market from America, where it had been available for a number of years. This was a bright blue liquid filled soft gelatin capsule formulation of diphenhydramine intended for use as a mild hypnotic. Very rapidly, drug misusers in Glasgow recognised its injection potential (similar to the early formulations of temazepam). The company concerned reacted responsibly and voluntarily removed the product from the market initially in Glasgow, followed by Scotland, and then the entire UK, once the abuse potential was highlighted to them. This incident has been reported in full (Roberts *et al.*, 1999).

Sympathomimetics

Many proprietary cough and cold remedies contain sympathomimetic drugs. These include pseudoephedrine, ephedrine, phenylpropanolamine and phenylephrine. These compounds are structurally related to amphetamine and in high doses are stimulants and appetite depressants. As such they are liable to misuse and products which combine these drugs with antihistamines have been particularly notorious. Although there is little evidence of increased physical ability, they have all been banned by the International Olympic Committee (see below). Likewise, they are not effective in producing prolonged weight loss.

Large doses can produce euphoria and pleasant changes in perception, although in some, especially the very young, these can be manifested as nightmares. Psychosis may result from excessive use of sympathomimetics, especially ephedrine. The symptoms usually resolve once the agent is removed, but long-term psychiatric problems may occur. In some countries pseudoephedrine is used as a precursor in the manufacture of methamphetamine. Pharmacists therefore have to be vigilant with regard to sales of pseudoephedrine-containing products.

Volatile substances

Pharmacists should also be aware of the abuse potential of non-medicinal products which contain volatile solvents (pharmacologically these act as depressants). It is illegal under the Intoxicating Substances Supply Act, 1985, for shopkeepers to sell such products in the knowledge that they were to be misused. However, this has been very difficult to prove in court. Almost any product which contains solvent or propellants can be inhaled, but in pharmacies the most likely are PR spray (Pain Relief Spray, an aerosol which contains propellant only), deodorant and hair sprays, and plaster and nail varnish removers. Pharmacists should ensure adequate training of all of their staff about this issue. Some pharmacists may receive requests to purchase large volumes of specific solvents. These may be required for purification of street drugs. Some ketones and nitriles are used as starting materials in the synthesis of amphetamine-type drugs (so called designer drugs). In many cases the supply of such materials is controlled. It goes without saying that surgical and methylated spirits can be drunk by alcoholics, who cannot afford even the cheapest alcoholic beverages. Obviously, in such cases, the adulterants added to make them unfit for consumption will cause toxicity, most importantly blindness.

A related group of products, which still seems to be freely available OTC although not from pharmacies, are "poppers". These are sold from sex shops and other outlets in small quantities up to 20 ml as room deodorisers and consist of amyl or butyl nitrites. Amyl nitrite was used by previous generations in the treatment of angina and, in pharmaceutical form, was available in small glass phials (vitrellae), which were crushed to release the drug causing a popping noise – hence the slang name. Butyl nitrite has never been used therapeutically. Sales of these products are restricted under the Medicines Act 1968, making sale from sex shops illegal, but prosecutions have been a rarity. In a case brought by the Royal Pharmaceutical Society, a sex shop owner was found guilty, but fined only a nominal amount and the RPSGB was not even awarded costs (Anon, 1996). Although at one time poppers were associated with homosexual practices because of their muscle relaxant properties, they are now widely used in the club scene as an alternative to ecstasy (Wills, 1997). In fact they are the most used drug after cannabis by the 16–29-year-old group according to the latest British Crime Survey carried out in March–April 1998 (Ramsay and Partridge, 1999).

Analgesics

Prolonged use of OTC analgesic remedies containing multiple antipyretic analgesics with caffeine and/or codeine is well known. Where such daily use extends over years, analgesic nephropathy is a potential consequence (De Broe and Elseviers, 1998). This is a progressive disease of the kidney characterised by renal papillary necrosis and chronic interstitial nephritis. It is not reversible and is treated by dialysis and renal transplantation. Originally, it was considered that phenacetin was the cause, since this drug was a component of most proprietary multi-component analgesic preparations available worldwide in the 1950s and 60s. Many countries, including the UK and Australia, removed phenacetin from the market during the 1970s. This has reduced, but not eliminated the incidence of analgesic nephropathy. Prescott (1982) has challenged this view of phenacetin being the "sole culprit" and suggested that the combination of analgesic agents was the key factor. It may be that a minor metabolite of phenacetin or paracetamol (acetaminophen, INN) is responsible, but this metabolite is potentiated by concomitant use of other drugs, in particular aspirin. Hence countries such as Australia have banned OTC sale of analgesic mixtures (Nanra, 1993), which has lead to a greater reduction in kidney disease. Pharmacists should where possible only recommend single component analgesic preparations for short-term use. Patients suspected of long-term misuse of these preparations should be counselled and advised to see their GP.

Laxatives

Two kinds of laxative abusers are recognised. Many older women are obsessed with ensuring a daily bowel movement and as such use stimulant laxatives (such as senna or bisacodyl) on a daily basis, despite the fact that they have no symptoms of constipation. Such use should be discouraged, although this group are not seen as a serious problem. A younger group, again mainly female, are more problematic. These people are obsessed with their weight and assume incorrectly that by taking stimulant laxatives they can decrease the calorific content of food they have eaten. This drug use itself can lead to serious consequences, such as hypokalaemia. However, this behaviour pattern can also reveal an underlying eating disorder such as anorexia and/or bulimia. Consequently they should be encouraged to discuss their anxieties with their doctor, although of course many will not face up to their real problems.

Products used in preparation of injected illicit drugs

Pharmacists need to keep alert regarding the misuse potential of some surprising products. Citric and ascorbic acid powders are used to make heroin more water soluble, so that it can be filtered from less soluble adulterants in street heroin prior to injecting. Although these products are available through outlets other than pharmacies, sales through pharmacies are covered by the paraphernalia clause of the Misuse of Drugs Act 1971 (see Chapter 9) and as such must not be sold to known or suspected drug users. However, many drug agencies are unaware of this and are perplexed by pharmacists' refusal to sell. There are now signs of a relaxation of attitudes by the authorities.

However, recently in South Wales, concern has been expressed over increases in requests for Ashton and Parsons infants' powders® (Ranshaw, personal communication). Apparently drug dealers find the wrappers ideal for distributing street drugs, using the powder itself to "cut" their supplies. A similar situation occurs elsewhere with Askit Powders®. Menthol cones, menthol crystals and vapour rubs cause vasodilation of the peripheral blood vessels and hence lead to rapid cooling. This property is used to prevent overheating by ecstasy users.

Nicotine replacement therapy

A new phenomenon since the availability of most nicotine replacement therapy (NRT) products as OTC medicines is the prospect of creating "NRT addicts". In fact this fear is probably one of the reasons which has limited the enthusiasm of some pharmacists to recommend this treatment as a useful adjunct to smoking cessation programmes. However, NRT supplies nicotine to the body without the harmful effects of the smoke itself. Hence moving a "cigarette addict" to an "NRT addict" has major benefits in a harm minimisation context. It is not yet clear whether very long-term use of NRT will become a real issue, which may have some specific toxic sequelae (other than the known toxicity of nicotine). In the meantime, pharmacists should use the effective products available to them, along with counselling, to assist smokers to quit. The situation with pregnant smokers is problematic at present. No NRT product is yet licensed for use by pregnant women. The Government has made this one of their key smoking research priorities and the outcome of this research is keenly awaited (Department of Health, 1998).

OTC DRUGS AND SPORTS

The misuse of drugs in sport continues to receive widespread media coverage, particularly after an elite athlete fails a drugs test and is banned from their sport. This has resulted in most sporting bodies taking the whole issue much more seriously, so that even at fairly low levels of amateur sport the regulations of the International Olympic Committee Medical Commission have been implemented. Hence pharmacists may be faced with questions of how to treat specific conditions without raising the risk of the patient being banned from their sport. The prohibited classes of substances have been widely publicised and consist of stimulants, narcotic analgesics, anabolic agents, diuretics as well as peptide and glycoprotein hormones (Bird and Verroken, 1998). From this list pharmacists offering OTC medication need only be concerned with stimulants, particularly caffeine, ephedrine and other sympathomimetic amines, as well as morphine, which is available in small quantities in a number of preparations. Codeine was originally in the banned list, but has been removed now. This provides a number of options for moderately strong OTC pain preparations. Non-steroidal anti-inflammatory drugs have not been banned and can also be used topically. Most sports cite a specific level, which must not be exceeded for caffeine. This allows moderate use of tea, coffee and other beverages, but caffeine-containing drug products should be avoided. Several individual sports, such as motor racing, archery, fencing, football and rugby have banned alcohol and marijuana. Some OTC liquid preparations contain a small percentage of alcohol in the diluent.

An emerging and highly lucrative market is the sale of vitamin and mineral supplements to athletes, including an increasing range of herbal remedies. Genuine vitamins and minerals are permitted, but care must be taken because some products may contain banned substances such as ephedrine or steroids. Likewise, some proprietary herbal remedies may be spiked with steroids. Many plants, such as chinese ephra, contain ephedrine naturally. Various amino acid mixtures are used, largely in response to the latest fad. However, creatine has become extremely widely used. This is stored in the skeletal muscle in the form of creatine phosphate, which provides a source of energy for short-term high energy activity, such as weight lifting or sprinting. Due to the difficulty in identifying exogenous creatine from endogenous, it has not been banned at present.

HOW SHOULD PHARMACISTS RESPOND TO MISUSERS OF OTC PRODUCTS?

The earlier discussions have classified three types of misusers of OTC products as follows:

(a) people who have become "addicted" following initial legitimate use of the products.
(b) people who are experimenting with OTC products seeking "kicks".
(c) people who are seeking a substitute for "hard drugs", when these are unavailable to them.

It may be possible to try and prevent a patient becoming a "type a misuser" by exerting vigilance over the amount of such a product sold and frequency of purchase. Furthermore, clear instructions should be given on the use of these products to "bona fide" patients. Leaflets on appropriate use of each class of OTC product, written in plain English, may be useful to back up such discussions. On the other hand, pharmacists may have little option but to restrict availability of products to customers in groups B and C, where they have suspected or clearly identified misuse. Indeed from time to time the RPSGB has suggested that certain items are removed from open view of customers and stored in the back of the shop. This was the solution most often cited by Northumberland and Northern Ireland pharmacists (see above). Closer working relationships between pharmacists and GPs, who are treating patients who are dependent on harder drugs, would give rise to opportunities to talk to the patient and possibly discuss the situation with the GP. Clearly there is a confidentiality issue here, but if a three-way contract between the user, the doctor and the pharmacist has been established, then it would be in the patient's interest. It would appear that drug users do not usually talk about their OTC use of drugs to GPs and drug workers trying to help them.

Ethical guidance within pharmacy

The RPSGB has over the years developed guidance for pharmacists in the form of the Code of Ethics. As stated above, the first Principle in this Code is that "a pharmacist's prime concern must be for the welfare of both the patient and other members of the public" (RPSGB, 1999). As long ago as 1939, the Council of the RPSGB issued a Statement Upon Matters of Professional Conduct, which directed that pharmacists should not sell any drug or medicine "notoriously capable of being used to gratify addiction or for other abusive purposes" (Appelbe, 1992). This statement has been modified over the years to its current form, which is included as an "Obligation" in the expansion of the first principle quoted above: "A pharmacist must exercise professional judgement to prevent the supply of unnecessary and excessive quantities of medicines and other products, particularly those which are liable to misuse, or which are claimed to depress appetite, prevent absorption of food or reduce body fluid" (RPSGB, 1999).

Further guidance is given to this obligation with regard to OTC medicines as follows: "Some over-the-counter medicines and non-medicinal products are liable to be misused, which in this context usually means (a) consumption over a lengthy period and/or (b) consumption of doses substantially higher than recommended. Requests for such products should be dealt with personally by the pharmacist and sale should be refused if it is apparent that the purchase is not for a genuine medicinal purpose or if the frequency of purchase suggests overuse. A pharmacist should not attempt on his own to control a misuser's habit, but should liaise with bodies such as drug misuse clinics in any local initiative to assist misusers." There is a further page in *Medicines, Ethics and Practice: A Guide for Pharmacists* devoted to substances of misuse, which lists many of the products (RPSGB, 1999).

Despite such clear cut advice and guidance, some pharmacists have been found guilty by the Statutory Committee of the RPSGB of misconduct for selling excessive quantities of codeine linctus, Phensedyl® (which contained codeine and promethazine), or similar products. A few years ago Appelbe (1992) concluded that the problem was becoming more widespread, with only one case heard prior to 1965 (in 1952), seven in the decade 1966/75, 16 between 1976 and 1985, but 20 in the next five years to 1990. However, the problem may have peaked, since John *et al.* (1999) could only find eight cases reported in the *Pharmaceutical Journal* during the period 1990–1998 which related to "uncontrolled supply of drugs of misuse".

In a case heard in 1992, a community pharmacist in London had sold over 600 litres of codeine linctus in a six-month period in 1990 (Anon, 1992). He claimed to be trying to help people give up drugs by reducing their supply of the linctus, but he had kept no records and had not discussed the matter with other local pharmacists or general medical practitioners. The Chairman of the RPSGB's Statutory Committee, Mr Gary Flather QC, concluded that "...This sort of attitude is simply wholly unacceptable. We cannot have pharmacists acting on their own without reference to any other persons such as medical men, clinics, or indeed to any other person experienced in this field..." (Anon, 1992). He then directed that the name of this pharmacist be removed from the Register of Pharmaceutical Chemists. A similar fate resulted to pharmacists in virtually all other cases.

WHAT ELSE CAN COMMUNITY PHARMACISTS DO?

Most community pharmacists are deeply disturbed by the rise in misuse of drugs and are extremely conscious of the misuse potential of this type of product. Their response to reminders from the RPSGB over the years, accompanied by an increasing demand from certain members of the public, has been to remove the main "culprit" products from the shelves in the public area of their premises. In most pharmacies, codeine linctus, and some other preparations, are stocked only in the dispensary (if at all) and sold only rarely to customers with "genuine" coughs. The usual ploy is to say that they are "out of stock" and recommend pholcodine linctus instead. (This product is an effective cough suppressant, but seems to have a low misuse potential.) One result of this has been a move by misusers away from the traditional products to an ever increasing range of "substitutes" or the exhaustive search by the misuser for a "friendly" pharmacist who is willing to oblige. Such pharmacists are likely to be deluged with customers. In the case cited above, it appeared that the pharmacist was serving 30 to 40 people per day with codeine linctus.

Alternative approaches

For those who have no interest in quitting their OTC misuse, their activities are often covert and may not be known to the pharmacist. However, there may be many people who knowingly or unwittingly misuse OTCs who could be helped by the pharmacist. As previously described, one way of dealing with the problem in the short term is simply to remove the items from show and refuse to sell them. However, two questions have to be posed:

> "Where will the misuser turn to seek other (perhaps more dangerous) supplies of the drug or an alternative, if no pharmacist is prepared to sell the products requested?"

> "What is the harm to the individual and society, if the individual consumes on a regular basis products such as codeine linctus, which have been sold openly and legally by a pharmacist?"

It is clearly very difficult to answer these questions definitively, since very little research has been carried out in these areas. Many pharmacists feel that some of the misusers they see (especially older persons) have become dependent on products which were initially purchased for real health reasons.

Some community pharmacists may want to help patients who appear to be dependent on OTC medicines, but are otherwise not part of the drug misuse scene. The official guidelines on the clinical management of drug misuse (Departments of Health, 1999) have been published primarily for general practitioners and contain very little advice on management of dependence of this type of product. In the past, some of these patients have been offered methadone maintenance through local drug agencies. This seems inappropriate, although the earlier Government guidelines for the management of drug misuse (Department of Health, 1991) have included a table of methadone equivalents, including an equivalent for codeine.

Practical help to such patients is a role that should be encouraged in order to reduce the chance of some misusers graduating into more serious problems. But how can community pharmacists offer a service which is acceptable to the ethical constraints of the profession? Clearly they must not act alone. This is the main criticism laid out in Statutory Committee rulings (e.g. Anon, 1992). The recommendations for GPs are that "a multidisciplinary approach to treatment is essential" (Departments of Health, 1999). How then can local liaison best be organised in order to help such patients?

A hypothetical scenario has been put forward by the author to various drug misuse groups and published in the pharmaceutical press (Temple, 1996). This suggests that the pharmacist maintains the therapy of the patient, through allowing controlled access to the preferred drug product, following a signed contract with the patient, which allows for full collaboration with the local community drug team (CDT) and/or GP and extensive record keeping. Unfortunately to date it has not been possible to examine this suggestion in a pilot scheme.

However, in the meantime, there is a real need for pharmacists to maintain closer contact generally with GPs and community drug teams (CDTs) in order to discuss issues relating to OTC drug misuse in a generic way. Indeed it would seem to be entirely compatible with the policy statement issued by the Royal Pharmaceutical Society in August 1991, which included the comment: "Liaison with medical practitioners and community drug teams is essential to ensure a co-ordinated approach to the provision of services to drug misusers in each locality" (Anon, 1991), although this statement did not mention services with respect to sale of OTC preparations. This would create the right atmosphere locally to offer some positive help to an OTC misuser who seeks help or who accepts the need to deal with a problem that has been highlighted by the pharmacist. Although pharmacists by and large are not trained in counselling techniques, they could spend some time with the drug user discussing their problem with them and trying to assist them to identify some potential solutions. With their permission, it would be possible to discuss their specific case with others, although patient confidentiality must be respected. Working with a patient and a CDT in this way would create an ideal means of specific training for the pharmacist, who would be better adapted to deal with future patients. The clinical psychologist or equivalent could well act as a mentor in such a scenario.

Creating new and improved opportunities to discuss the local drug misuse scene would have additional benefits. For instance it should be feasible to establish an early warning system through the Local Pharmaceutical Committee and/or CDT when there is indication of a misuse of a specific product in the locality. A good example of this was discussed above in the case of Sleepia® in Glasgow.

CONCLUSIONS

A range of issues relating to misuse of OTC preparations of relevance to the community pharmacist have been covered in this chapter. This includes specific interactions with users of hard drugs covered in other chapters, but also introduces a range of other clients in the pharmacy, from those primarily dependent on OTC products, either through initial bona fide use or as a deliberate act of experimentation, to those seeking advice to avoid accusations of cheating from sporting bodies. In all cases, the pharmacist is recommended to maintain close contacts with other professionals in the area, both to share knowledge as part of continuing professional development and to better help a specific client.

REFERENCES

Anon (1991). Pharmaceutical services for drug misusers. *Pharmaceutical Journal*, 247, 223.

Anon (1992). Excessive codeine linctus sales lead to striking off. *Pharmaceutical Journal*, 249, 714.

Anon (1996). Society wins 'poppers' case at a price. *Pharmaceutical Journal*, 256, 883.

Appelbe GE (1992). *The Control of Discipline in the Pharmaceutical Profession*. PhD. thesis, University of Wales.

Ball K, Wilde M (1989). OTC medicines misuse in West Cumbria. *Pharmaceutical Journal*, 242, 40.

Bird J, Verroken M (1998). *Competitors and Officials Guide to Drugs and Sport*. United Kingdom Sports Council, London.

De Broe ME, Elseviers MM (1998). Analgesic Nephropathy. *New England Journal of Medicine*, 338, 446–452.

Department of Health (1991). *Drug Misuse and Dependence – Guidelines on Clinical Management*, HMSO, London.

Department of Health (1998). *Smoking Kills – A White Paper on Tobacco*, Department of Health, London.

Departments of Health (1999). *Drug Misuse and Dependence – Guidelines on Clinical Management*. The Stationery Office, London.

Hughes GF, McElnay JC, Hughes CM, McKenna P (1999). Abuse/misuse of non-prescription drugs. *Pharmacy World and Science*, 21, 251–255.

John DE, Angell RN, Genner S, Hussain MZ (1999). A descriptive study of reasons for appearing before, and outcomes of, Statutory Committee hearings. *Pharmaceutical Journal (supplement)*, 263, R48.

Nanra RS (1993). Analgesic nephropathy in the 1990s – an Australian perspective. *Kidney International (supplement)*, 42, S86–S92.

Paxton R, Chapple P (1996). Misuse of over-the-counter medicines: A survey in one English county. *Pharmaceutical Journal*, 256, 313–315.

Prescott LF (1982). Analgesic Nephropathy: a reassessment of the role of phenacetin and other analgesics. *Drugs*, 23, 75–149.

Ramsay M, Partridge S (1999). *Drug Misuse Declared in 1998: results from the British Crime Survey*, Home Office Research Study 197, Home Office, London.

Roberts K, Gruer L, Gilhooly T (1999). Misuse of diphenhydramine soft gelatine capsules (Sleepia): a cautionary tale from Glasgow. *Addiction*, 94, 1575–1578.

RPSGB (1999). *Medicines, Ethics and Practice: A Guide for Pharmacists. No. 22, July 1999*, The Royal Pharmaceutical Society of Great Britain, London.

Temple DJ (1996). Harm-reduction OTC. *Chemist and Druggist*, 245, 730–731.

Wills S (1993). Drugs and Substance Misuse: Over-the-counter Products. *Pharmaceutical Journal*, 251, 807–810.

Wills S (1997). *Drugs of Abuse*, The Pharmaceutical Press, London.

14

Providing health care for drug users

Sile O'Connor

INTRODUCTION

Drug users have the same rights to health care as other people. Furthermore, they have health care needs that are likely to exceed their age-matched norm. Many drug users are not in contact with structured drug treatment programmes, either because they have yet to reach the point where they need or want to address their problem drug use or because they have chosen to treat their addiction without using prescribed drugs. Although not in touch with specialist drug services during this time, drug users could use, and certainly could benefit from, the health care services provided by their local community pharmacy.

Other pharmacy customers are generally unaware of the drug user's need for pharmacy-based health care services, possibly with the exception of supervised consumption of methadone. This means that drug users can use these services in their local community pharmacy without coming under scrutiny from other customers, and without experiencing the possible stigmatisation associated with attendance at specialist services concerned only with the drug user.

Community pharmacies offer many health care services to their drug-using clientele. Firstly, drug users may use the community pharmacy-based services specifically designed for them – primarily methadone dispensing services, the sale or supply of injecting equipment, accompanied by advice on the disposal of used equipment and safer injecting practice and needle exchange facilities. These services are discussed above in Chapters 9, 10, 11 and 12.

The community pharmacy provides many generic health care services which are also beneficial to drug users, and these include:

- dispensing and supply of, and advice on, prescribed and "over-the-counter" medicines
- health promotion information and preventative advice on all aspects of personal health and well-being
- sale and supply of health care products
- referral of the patient to a GP, dentist or other health care professional for more specialist care and treatment
- advice on emergency situations.

The following sections outline some of these services.

ADVICE ON MEDICINES
Dispensing, supply and advice on prescribed and "over-the-counter" medicines
The community pharmacist is familiar with all prescribed drugs and "over-the-counter" medicines (see Chapter 13), and with the interactions and side-effects associated with them. For example many drugs cause drowsiness or impair co-ordination, particularly if taken in conjunction with methadone. In addition, some drug users may be receiving antiviral drugs for the management of HIV, and many of these interact with methadone, as do drugs used to treat tuberculosis, a condition now becoming more common among many drug users who sleep rough. A guide to drugs which interact with methadone can be found in the Government's 1999 Clinical Guidelines on the management for drug misuse (Departments of Health, 1999).

The new methadone patient
Whether or not methadone is being prescribed for long-term maintenance in patients unable or unwilling to achieve abstinence, or the patient is receiving a methadone detoxification, there will be an initial period during which the dose needs to be stabilised. Patients starting on methadone treatment should normally be on daily supervised instalment dispensing (Departments of Health, 1999), usually provided by the community pharmacist. This provides pharmacists with an opportunity to build up a professional relationship with new patients. Additionally, as methadone has a long half-life and therefore takes several days to reach steady state, pharmacists are in a position to monitor for signs of intoxication (in cases where the methadone dose may be too high or where patients are continuing to use other opiates "on top" of their methadone dose). Research has indicated that the first two weeks of methadone treatment are high-risk times for overdose (Caplehorn and Drummer, 1999). Pharmacists can also monitor for signs of withdrawal, where a patient's dose of methadone may not be high enough or where, for example, concomitant medication may increase or decrease methadone clearance and hence cause intoxication or withdrawal. In either case, a good professional relationship between the pharmacist and prescribing doctor will ensure that such information is fed back in order to maximise the safety and care of the patient. Pharmacists who are part of formal shared care arrangements for drug users will find that issues around confidentiality will be resolved as the patient will be aware that the pharmacist is part of the care team and as such will be sharing information in the context of the care of the patient.

Detoxification
Patients who are detoxifying from opioids may be prescribed opioid substitutes such as buprenorphine and methadone in reducing doses over a period of time which may be several weeks to months. In other cases, patients may be prescribed lofexidine, a centrally-acting alpha-2 adrenergic agonist, which suppresses some of the withdrawal symptoms caused by an overproduction of noradrenaline. These patients may also require further symptomatic treatment of symptoms such as diarrhoea and pain, and will receive additional prescriptions from their doctor for such medicines. Pharmacists may also find themselves dispensing reducing doses of other drugs such as diazepam for patients on a benzodiazepines withdrawal, and again support and encouragement are essential.

The role of the pharmacist does not end with the dispensing of such medications. Support and encouragement are key factors in any detoxification, either when patients are succeeding or when they are finding the detoxification difficult. Pharmacists involved in shared care arrangements may also find that they have the opportunity to feed back on a patient's progress at regular intervals.

Opioid maintenance therapy

For patients who are unable or unwilling to reduce their opioid intake, or who are not ready to achieve and maintain abstinence, maintenance treatment is an option. The most commonly prescribed drug for this in the UK is methadone, usually as an oral liquid and buprenorphine has recently been licenced in the UK for the management of opioid dependence. For such patients, the pharmacist has an opportunity to build patient–pharmacist relationships in which they can provide a variety of primary health care services and health promotion messages which are discussed later in this chapter. However, they can also monitor patients for changes in behaviour, being alert to signs such as deterioration in a patient's appearance, an increase in alcohol intake or even a change in the time of day when a patient collects their medication. A discussion with the patient may lead to an opportunity for the pharmacist to liaise with other members of the care team. As with all prescriptions for methadone, whether for detoxification or maintenance, the pharmacist should be vigilant regarding several missed doses, which could lead to a fall in the patient's tolerance making their usual dose of methadone potentially toxic, or to patients intoxicated with alcohol or other drugs, where concomitant use of methadone poses a risk of overdose. Many local areas have specific guidelines and protocols for managing such incidents, but pharmacists would be wise to discuss these issues with prescribers and set up mutually agreed protocols of which patients are informed.

Safe storage of medicine in the home

Community pharmacists should make their methadone patients aware of the dangers associated with the accidental ingestion of medicines by children or opiate naïve individuals, and advise patients on safe storage. Leaflets on the safe storage of medicines are available in many parts of the UK and Ireland. In the UK, methadone must be dispensed in child-resistant packaging. This is an important safety measure, given the lack of caution evident in the storage arrangements used by many drug users (Binchy *et al.*, 1994; Calman *et al.*, 1996). Other issues around safety with regard to methadone centre around the way in which drug users measure out daily doses of their methadone, when it has been dispensed in large instalments, e.g. a week's supply at once. A study in Ireland noted that many drug users use a variety of ways to measure out their methadone, including babies' bottles (Harkin *et al.*, 1999). Obviously this poses some risk to children if bottles are not adequately rinsed. Pharmacists can help to prevent this by ensuring patients have suitable measuring cups and are advised on the dangers of accidental overdose in small children.

HEALTH PROMOTION INFORMATION AND PREVENTATIVE ADVICE
Nutrition

The nutritional status of drug users is often poor, due to factors such as a chaotic lifestyle, lack of resources and ill health. One study showed that one quarter of a treatment sample had not eaten a cooked meal during the previous 72 hours and those who consumed larger amounts of alcohol ate less frequently (Best *et al.*, 1998). Problematic drug use is often associated with erratic eating and sleeping, reducing drug users' natural reserves and diminishing their immune system. Chronic use of heroin or alcohol, or short-term heavy use or "bingeing" with cocaine or stimulants can cause drug users' health to be seriously compromised.

During periods of chronic or heavy use or during withdrawal, drug users may experience rapid weight loss, mineral and vitamin deficiency, reduced muscle mass and severe dehydration. If this physical state is coupled with an underlying systemic problem, the drug user is ultimately likely to need in-patient treatment. Once the drug user's health is compromised, opportunistic infections, such as bronchitis or minor abscesses, can rapidly progress to pneumonia or septicaemia. It is vital that the community pharmacist works to ensure the drug user stays healthy by offering nutritional advice and encouraging a balanced diet. Conversely, drug users who stabilise on methadone, or begin to reduce or control their drug use, may begin to gain weight. Community pharmacists can advise these patients on eating healthily, with a reduced sugar and fat intake, to avoid this weight gain being instrumental in triggering relapse to chaotic drug use. Patients with chronic infections such as hepatitis and tuberculosis may require special dietary advice.

As well as general information on balanced nutrition and ideal body weights, drug-using patients may need specific dietary information including details of vitamin-rich foods, high-fibre diets to reduce chronic constipation due to long-term opiate use, and often associated with haemorrhoids, and immune-strengthening foods to fight infection, improve healing and slow the progression of disease.

There are circumstances where the community pharmacist should refer the drug user for specialist nutritional advice. Chronic alcohol abuse commonly results in severe vitamin and mineral deficiencies. This, coupled with poor absorption, may lead to a dangerous reduction in vitamins B, C and K (Dodds, 1991). Where chronic alcohol abuse is suspected, the pharmacist can refer the patient for immediate medical attention. Opiate users who become pregnant should be advised to contact local ante-natal services, since they commonly suffer from anaemia and various vitamin deficiencies including B6, folate and thiamine (Siney *et al.*, 1995) (see below).

Cigarette smoking

Studies of drug users in treatment have shown that the majority of drug users smoke cigarettes – in one study 93% smoked, with a mean intake of 18 cigarettes per day (Best *et al.*, 1998), and a significant proportion also smoke cannabis. The impact of smoking on health in an otherwise healthy individual is considerable and pharmacists are in a position to advise on smoking cessation.

Dental care

Drug users have been found to have poorer oral health and to use dental services less frequently than an age and gender-matched non-drug-using population (Sheridan *et al.*, 2001) and anecdotally methadone users report problematic side-effects such as dental problems. Methadone reduces the production of saliva, which has a protective role in the mouth, so those on methadone may have associated aggravation of dental decay. However, research shows that drug users who have never been prescribed methadone are just as likely to experience poor dental health as those on methadone, so it appears that methadone may exacerbate pre-existing dental problems, rather than causing new ones (Lewis, 1990). Smoking heroin or nicotine can stain the teeth, and drug users who apply cocaine powder to their gums may also experience localised dental damage (Preston, 1996).

As drug users stabilise on methadone and especially when they start to detoxify from opiates, they often report experiencing dental pain. This is probably because they have a reduced awareness of dental degeneration during chronic or chaotic drug use due to the excellent pain-relieving properties of heroin and methadone (Preston, 1996). Indeed, this pain may trigger relapse to illicit drug use. Therefore, it is essential that drug users address their dental health as part of any stabilisation or detoxification programme. In addition to supplying opiate-free, over-the-counter, anti-inflammatory painkillers for immediate use, where necessary the community pharmacist can encourage the drug-using customer to attend a dentist for a full dental examination.

Vein damage and wound management
Where drug users are actively involved in injecting practice, they may experience cuts and sores, cellulitis, recurrent abscesses and ulcers, at the most frequently used injection sites. If a patient's wound is deep, seriously infected or where the pharmacist is unsure, a referral should be made to a GP or Accident and Emergency unit. If appropriate, advice can be given on choice of dressings, frequency of dressing change and the use of antiseptic applications. If left untreated, the patient is at risk of developing septicaemia and consequent future health problems, for example bacterial endocarditis or renal complications.

Where the drug user is experiencing regular abscesses or ulcers, the community pharmacist, in addition to referring for treatment, can give basic safer injecting advice such as alternating injecting sites in order to reduce the incidence of infection and supply clean injecting equipment (see Chapter 10).

Injecting drug users are at risk of developing deep vein thrombosis (DVT), most commonly in the lower limbs. A number of factors increase the risk of DVT, such as injecting into the femoral vein, being overweight, smoking and lack of exercise. When DVT is suspected, the drug user should be referred immediately for medical attention. Continued injecting into the same vein can also cause veins to collapse, and after many years of injecting, it is common for drug users to have problems accessing veins.

Establishing or recovering sleep patterns
Many drug users totally lack a normal sleep pattern, which is often difficult to re-establish and leaves them psychologically frustrated and physically exhausted. Sleep is essential if the drug user is to recover health and well-being, and gradually regain control over life. Because of their history of dependence, the use of psychoactive or habit-forming prescribed medication is not recommended for many drug users. However, there are a number of strategies which can be employed to aid sleep and the pharmacist can provide advice on this. The community pharmacist can encourage the patient to exercise during the day, employ various relaxation techniques, eat healthily and establish a regular routine lifestyle. Other advice can include the use of

aromatherapy oils which promote relaxation, such as lavender and clary sage, and a reduction in caffeine intake and the use of herbal teas which promote sleep such as chamomile. Herbal remedies may also be advised, but pharmacists may wish to check with the drug company or local drug information services about any interactions between these products and prescribed or illicit drugs.

Complementary medicines can also be employed, for example, to raise energy levels or feelings of well-being, for relaxation purposes, and to improve self-esteem. Remedies such as acupuncture and techniques such as yoga and massage are particularly useful.

If a normal sleeping pattern still does not return, a referral for a further medical or psychiatric assessment might be appropriate, since this may be indicative of underlying depression, anxiety, bipolar (manic/depressive) or other mental illness. The community pharmacist will need to assess the circumstances to determine whether such a referral is necessary.

Support and encouragement

Although the needs of drug users with more complex psychological problems are discussed later, many drug users will suffer from poor self-esteem and feel marginalised. The positive impact of encouragement and support should not be underestimated. When patients seem to be making positive health gains, or where they have secured a job, for example, pharmacists can recognise this with positive feedback. Furthermore, pharmacists can help to motivate patients with regard to making such changes. A more detailed discussion on the role of the "talking therapies" can be found in Chapter 15, and pharmacists may wish to undertake formal training in some of these techniques.

BLOOD-BORNE VIRUSES AND OTHER INFECTIOUS DISEASES
Testing, vaccination and advice

Although there are no vaccines against HIV or hepatitis C, many other infectious diseases which are blood-borne or sexually transmitted can be prevented. While a certain level of public awareness of the transmission routes and symptoms of HIV has been achieved, and infection may have slowed, the seroprevalences of hepatitis B and C remain worryingly high among the drug using population. The seroprevalence of hepatitis C is estimated at between 60% and 80%, and for hepatitis B around 20–60% (Gossop *et al.*, 1994; Rhodes *et al.*, 1996; Best *et al.*, 1999).

Hepatitis B is also sexually transmitted, and hence is not limited to the drug-using population, but also to their sexual partners. Furthermore, over 30% of those with acute hepatitis B infection do not have identifiable risk factors. In response to recommendations from the World Health Assembly and the World Health Organisation, more than 80 countries had included hepatitis B vaccine as a routine part of their infant or adolescent immunisation programmes by 1996 (van Damme *et al.*, 1997). Each year one million people die from hepatitis B, and there are 350 million chronic carriers world-wide (WHO, 1996). Because the hepatitis B virus is about 100 times more infective than HIV, the cleaning techniques used for injecting equipment which are adequate to avoid HIV transmission are not necessarily sufficient to prevent the spread of the hepatitis B virus among drug users, and it is essential that drug users are offered vaccination against hepatitis B. In a recent study of drug agencies in England and Wales, less than 30% routinely provided hepatitis B testing and vaccination (Winstock *et al.*, 2000).

Where hepatitis C is present, its rate of progression may be greatly increased by subsequent infection with hepatitis B or A. Therefore dual vaccination against hepatitis A and B should be recommended to drug users who are hepatitis C positive (Vento *et al.*, 1998). The community pharmacist can play a role in informing drug-using customers of the availability of the hepatitis A and B vaccination, and encouraging them to be vaccinated.

The latest anti-retroviral drugs are very effective in reducing the progress of the HIV virus, and in practice, the sooner a positive diagnosis can be established, the better the prognosis for the patient (Palella *et al.*, 1998). Furthermore, hepatitis B is entirely preventable by vaccination. Therefore, drug users who have engaged in high risk behaviour (either sharing injecting equipment, injecting paraphernalia such as swabs, filters, water [see Chapter 9 for more details] or unprotected sexual activity) should be encouraged to consider being tested. Community pharmacists who are aware of injecting drug use in a customer may have the opportunity to discreetly enquire about their knowledge of their hepatitis B status, as drug users who are hepatitis B negative can be vaccinated against the disease.

Pharmacists can further support clients who have tested positive for HIV and hepatitis B and C. For example, patients with a stable lifestyle, who avoid alcohol and undergo drug therapy, can improve their prognoses. Community pharmacists should actively encourage hepatitis C positive drug-using patients to reduce their alcohol intake and link in regularly with hepatology services.

TUBERCULOSIS

The pharmacist can give the patient information about prescribed medication and encourage compliance with the prescribed dosage regimen. This is particularly important where the drugs involved have many associated side effects and where poor compliance may lead to resistance and reduced efficacy of treatment (Humma, 1996; Joint Tuberculosis Committee of the British Thoracic Society, 1998). Poor patient compliance can cause previously drug-susceptible bacteria to acquire resistance to one or more of the drugs being administered, resulting in secondary resistance (Humma, 1996). The pharmacist may further augment patient compliance by offering to supervise daily dosing on-site (Joint Tuberculosis Committee of the British Thoracic Society, 1998). Supervising the self-administration of other drug therapy on-site is particularly useful for patients who self-administer their methadone on-site at the pharmacy since some of these patients may be reluctant to take concurrent treatments which cause nausea, for fear of vomiting their methadone dose.

CONTRACEPTION AND SAFER SEX

Many drug and alcohol users, particularly those who are not engaged in treatment, have chaotic lifestyles. The absence of daily or monthly routine reduces the feasibility of family planning while disinhibition and altered sensory perception may raise the risk of exposure to sexually transmitted infection in this group.

The risks associated with unprotected sexual contact have been highly publicised, encouraging all members of the public to avoid disease transmission by using barrier contraceptives, and community pharmacists are well positioned to reinforce this safer sex message. Community pharmacists supply a variety of condoms and other "over-the-counter" contraceptive products in an accessible and anonymous setting, and can help the customer to choose a particular product depending on their needs and can also dispense prescriptions for prescribed contraceptives.

Community pharmacists should be aware that heavy or chronic use of opiates and other drugs, coupled with poor nutrition, means that female drug users may have irregular or absent periods (ISDD, 1992). The pharmacist can discreetly ensure the customer knows that this does not mean she is infertile and unable to conceive, and that she should take precautions, if necessary, to avoid pregnancy. Indeed, the female opiate user who successfully stabilises on methadone may be particularly at risk of unwanted pregnancy since her health may improve sufficiently for her to re-establish ovulation (even if without a regular menstrual cycle).

GROUPS WITH SPECIAL NEEDS
Pregnant drug users
Pregnant drug users may experience a great deal of anxiety. In addition to the usual worries created by the imminent responsibilities associated with parenthood, they may also worry about their child being taken into care if health workers find out about their drug use. (Drug use *per se* does not necessarily constitute a reason for a child to be taken into care). The importance of ante-natal care for the future health of the mother and the child has been strongly emphasised by the WHO (Rooney, 1992).

Pharmacists can advise on appropriate nutrition and folic acid intake during pregnancy, as well as trying to ensure that the drug-user has made contact with relevant health care services and is receiving ante-natal care.

Pregnancy is an event which prompts many females to want to stop using drugs. Many certainly express the desire to do so, and experience guilt if they continue to use (Siney, 1995). Referral to a drug agency is advised as methadone has been used safely in mothers who want to detoxify while pregnant (Finnegan *et al.*, 1991). A more cautious approach to detoxification is taken so as to keep to a minimum any withdrawal distress and consequent risk to the unborn child. However, detoxification is not always recommended as it can cause problems during the first and third trimesters. The most important treatment may be to stabilise a woman's drug use and reduce the risks to mother and baby of continued injecting drug use. Methadone should be prescribed in adequate doses to eliminate, as far as possible, any illicit drug use (Kaltenbach *et al.*, 1998). Research shows that women who attend treatment services generally have better ante-natal care and better health than drug-using women not in treatment, even if they are still using illicit drugs (Bately and Weissel, 1993). The community pharmacist can also advise about the impact of the use of legal and illegal drugs during pregnancy, including the use of alcohol and nicotine (Kline *et al.*, 1987), which have been associated with premature births and low birth-weights.

Post-natal support is also essential in maintaining health and well-being in both mother and child. It is common for post-natal women to attend the local community pharmacy for items such as nappy rash creams, and treatments for haemorrhoids or constipation and women on methadone may be transferred directly from the hospital to their GP and community pharmacy. Furthermore, specific advice on breast-feeding and drug use may be provided. Breast-feeding is contraindicated in HIV-positive women (Departments of Health, 1999) due to the risk of transmission of the virus from mother to baby.

Psychological and other mental health issues

The co-existence of mental health problems and drug and alcohol abuse is well documented (Hall and Farrell, 1997). Drug users may have mental health problems as a result of their drug use, or such problems may have pre-dated drug use. Furthermore, drug use may be a form of self-medication for mental health problems. However, it is often difficult to disentangle the relationship, and the fact that many drug users have mental health problems is often associated with poor integration of care. Drug users comprise a particularly vulnerable group, and a group that may have lost contact with formal health services. From the community pharmacy perspective, such patients may be more difficult to manage; however, the pharmacist is in a prime position to be able to refer such patients for more specialised care.

Studies have shown that those who are homeless or sleeping rough often have co-existing mental health and drug and alcohol problems (Rough Sleepers Unit, 1999). This group of individuals is likely to be out of contact with primary health and specialist health care, and may not have a GP. The community pharmacist may be the most viable contact with primary health care – perhaps their only contact. Pharmacists may be able to provide advice and help around a number of health issues such as wound care and nutrition. They are also in a position to help individuals engage with more specialised services.

SUMMARY

Most of the services discussed above will already be being offered to the whole community, and for drug users who do not wish to access specialist drug services, the availability of these services in a community pharmacy may be particularly important. Pharmacists should not underestimate the impact they can have on the health and psychological well-being of drug users, even if they are unwilling to dispense drugs such as methadone or enter into formal needle exchange arrangements. The care of drug users, as with all patients, extends far beyond their medical diagnosis, and a holistic approach to care is encouraged.

Community pharmacists who are interested in developing their input into the health care of drug users need to establish good links with other local health care providers, so that they are aware of the services each of them provides and can offer comprehensive information on these services if required. Good links also ease the referral process, where necessary. The importance of the community pharmacy within the local network lies in its ability to provide many first line health care services in the absence of local specialist care.

Acknowledgement/Thanks to:

Noreen Geoghegan, Drugs & AIDS Service Maternity Liaison Nurse, E.H.B., Dr Shay Keating, Hepatology Specialist, Drugs & AIDS Service, E.H.B. and Orla Sheehan, National Medicines Information Centre, St James' Hospital, Dublin.

REFERENCES

Bately RG, Weissel K (1993). A 40-month follow-up of pregnant drug using women treated at Westmead Hospital. *Drug and Alcohol Review*, 12, 265–270.

Best D, Lehmann P, Gossop M, Harris J, Noble A, Strang J (1998). Eating too little, smoking and drinking too much: wider lifestyle problems among methadone maintenance patients. *Addiction Research*, 6, 489–498.

Best D, Noble A, Finch E, Gossop M, Sidwell C, Strang J (1999). Accuracy of perceptions of hepatitis B and C status: a cross sectional investigation of opiate addicts in treatment. *British Medical Journal*, 319, 290–291.

Binchy JM, Molyneux EM, Manning J (1994). Accidental ingestion of methadone by children in Merseyside. *British Medical Journal*, 308, 1335–1336.

Calman L, Finch E, Powis B, Strang J (1996). Only half of patients store methadone in safe place (letter). *British Medical Journal*, 313, 1481.

Caplehorn JR, Drummer OH (1999). Mortality associated with New South Wales methadone programs in 1994: lives lost and saved. *Medical Journal of Australia*, 170,104–109.

Departments of Health *et al.* (1999). *Drug Misuse and Dependence: Guidelines on Clinical Management*, The Stationery Office, London.

Dodds L (Ed) (1991). *Drugs in Use: clinical case studies for pharmacists*, Pharmaceutical Press, London, pp 88–89.

Finnegan LP, Hagan T, Kaltenbach KA (1991). Scientific foundation of clinical practice: Opiate use in pregnant women. *Bulletin of the New York Academy of Medicine*, 67, 223–239.

Gossop M, Powis B, Griffiths P, Strang J (1994). Multiple risk for HIV and hepatitis B infection among heroin users. *Drug and Alcohol Review*, 13, 293–300.

Hall W, Farrell M (1997). Co-morbidity of mental disorders with substance abuse. *British Journal of Psychiatry*, 171, 4–5.

Harkin K, Quinn C, Bradley F (1999). Storing methadone in babies' bottles puts young children at risk (letter). *British Medical Journal*, 318, 329.

Institute for the Study of Drug Dependence (1992). *Drugs, Pregnancy and Childcare: A Guide for Professionals.* ISDD, London.

Joint Tuberculosis Committee of the British Thoracic Society, BTS Guidelines (1998). Chemotherapy and management of tuberculosis in the United Kingdom: recommendations 1998. *Thorax*, 53, 536–548.

Kaltenbach K, Berghella V, Finnegan L (1998). Opioid dependence during pregnancy. Effects and Management. *Obstetrics and Gynecology Clinics of North America*, 25, 139–51.

Kline J, Stein Z, Hutzler M (1987). Cigarettes, alcohol and marijuana: varying associations with birthweight. *International Journal of Epidemiology*, 16, 44–51.

Lewis D (1990). Methadone and caries. *British Dental Journal*, 168, 349.

Palella FJ, Delaney KM, Moorman AC, Loveless MO, Fuhrer J, Satten GA, Aschmann DJ, Holmberg SD (1998). Declining morbidity and mortality among patients with advanced human immunodeficiency virus infection. HIV Outpatient Study Investigations. *New England Journal of Medicine*, 338, 853–860.

Preston A (Ed) (1996). *The Methadone Briefing.* ISDD, London, p. 50.

Rhodes T, Hunter GM, Stimson GV, Donoghoe MC, Noble A, Parry J, Chalmers C (1996). Prevalence of markers for hepatitis B virus and HIV-1 among drug injectors in London; injecting careers, positivity and risk behaviour. *Addiction*, 91, 1457–1467.

Rooney C (Ed) (1992). *Antenatal Care and Maternal Health: How Effective is it? A Review of the Evidence.* WHO, Geneva.

Rough Sleepers Unit (1999). *Coming in From the Cold: the Government's Strategy on Rough Sleeping.* Department of the Environment, Transport and the Regions (DETR), London.

Sheridan J, Aggleton M, Carson T (2001). Dental health and access to dental treatment: a comparison of drug users and non-drug users attending community pharmacies. *British Dental Journal*, 191, 453–457.

Siney C (Ed) (1995). *Obstetric Problems for Drug Users, The Pregnant Drug Addict.* The Royal College of Midwives, London, p. 25.

Siney C, Kidd M, Walkinshaw S, Morrison C, Manasse P (1995). Opiate dependency in pregnancy. *British Journal of Midwifery*, 3, 69–73.

van Damme P, Kane M, Meeheus A (on behalf of the Viral Hepatitis Prevention Board) (1997). Integration of hepatitis B vaccination into national immunisation programmes. *British Medical Journal*, 314, 1033–1077.

Vento S, Garafano T, Rensini C, Cainelli F, Casali F, Ghironzi G, Ferraro T, Concia E (1998). Fulminant hepatitis associated with hepatitis A virus superinfection in patients with chronic hepatitis C. *New England Journal of Medicine*, 338, 286–290.

WHO Viral Hepatitis Prevention Board (1996). *Prevention and Control of Hepatitis B in the Community.* WHO, Geneva.

Winstock A, Sheridan J, Lovell S, Farrell M, Strang J (2000). A National Survey of Hepatitis Testing and Vaccination Provision by Drug Services in England and Wales. *European Journal of Clinical Microbiology and Infectious Diseases*, 19, 823–828.

15

Psychology and addiction: the talking therapies

Tara Rado and Robert Hill

"If you have never been addicted, you can have no clear idea what it means to need junk with the addict's special need. You don't decide to be an addict. One morning you wake up sick and you're an addict"

(William Burroughs, 1977, p. xv).

Community pharmacists come into contact with people with many addictions – to nicotine, illicit drugs, alcohol for example, and this may be in the context of managing the addiction itself or the consequences of the addiction. Furthermore, they may also be involved in helping people to "quit" or modify an addiction, for example in the context of smoking cessation campaigns or through involvement with a needle and syringe exchange scheme. Talking to patients is normal practice for community pharmacists and the promotion of health is a key part of their role. As characterised by the WHO in the Ottawa Charter for Health promotion, health promotion is "the process of enabling people to increase their control over, and to improve, their health" and there is evidence that this type of health promotion is effective (Anderson and Blenkinsopp, 2001). Although research into the impact of pharmacy-related health promotion activities is limited, there is evidence that smoking cessation health promotion campaigns, for example, can be effective and acceptable (Sinclair *et al.*, 1995). Furthermore, the management of heroin addiction with methadone alone is not as effective as methadone plus psychosocial intervention, although methadone treatment alone brings about significant improvement in health and can also bring about behaviour change (Mattick *et al.*, 1998). Ball and Ross (1991) also noted that that counselling was believed to be the most important ingredient of the rehabilitative part of the methadone treatment programme, by both staff and clients in the study.

For many people it is hard to understand how someone can become addicted to drugs. Why can some people use drugs like cocaine or heroin in an apparently controlled manner for long periods of time, while others report that they became "addicted with the first dose"? Perhaps the fundamental problem with this question lies with the definition of an addiction. During the past thirty years the scientific understanding and public attitudes and beliefs towards what actually constitutes an addiction have radically changed. As a result of these changes, the word addiction is one of the most common words in everyday usage that can mean different things to different people.

In a recent review of theories of addiction, West (2001) cites the current definition of addiction as a behaviour over which an individual has impaired control with harmful consequences. This definition reflects the current move away from theories that merely focus on drug addiction, towards an all encompassing psychological theory that can account for a range of behaviours including excessive drinking, smoking, gambling, eating, sex and a diverse range of drugs including heroin, cocaine and cannabis (Orford, 2001). To date however, the majority of theories of addiction have focussed upon drug addiction. These theories have arisen as a result of research conducted in a wide range of research disciplines including behavioural pharmacology, social psychology, and cognitive psychology. However, for those clinical psychologists and health workers working in addiction, the most interesting and relevant theories of drug addiction are those that can lend themselves to clinical practice. Health workers have the greatest interest in those theories that aim to provide an account of why someone develops an addiction, what maintains it over time and most importantly, how it can best be treated.

The most popular approach among health workers working in addictions is to view compulsive drug seeking as the defining feature of drug addiction. The progression from experimental drug use to compulsive drug seeking is described as a continuum, where the drug user's behaviour is characterised by overwhelming involvement of the use of the drug, the securing of its supply, and a high tendency to relapse after withdrawal (Jaffe, 1975). Since compulsive drug seeking can result in a severe impairment in the drug user's quality of life in a vast range of ways, it is generally agreed that drug addiction may be considered a form of a psychiatric disorder. Specifically, it has recently been suggested that addiction may be considered to reflect a disorder of motivation (West, 2001).

The main psychological theories that can be linked to an evidenced-based treatment approach to drug addiction fall into one of three categories, although the dividing line is fine and is open to interpretation. Behavioural theories emphasise the important role of learning and conditioning processes in the development, maintenance and relapse of drug addiction. In contrast, cognitive theories highlight the role of drug-induced changes in mental state in the development, maintenance and relapse of drug addiction. Finally, derived from the principles of social-learning theory (Bandura, 1977), the cognitive-behavioural model of addiction accounts for both the behavioural and the cognitive approaches to addiction. The following sections will introduce these theories of drug addiction and provide a brief overview of the psychological interventions that have developed as a result of them.

BEHAVIOURAL THEORIES

"A clear white powder is not repulsive; it looks pure, it glitters, the pure white crystals sparkle like snow" (Anna Kavan, 1970, p. 101).

The premise of the behavioural approach is that addiction or the compulsive drug seeking behaviour thought to characterise an addiction is maintained as a result of the powerful reinforcing effects of a drug. This approach is built on the pivotal finding that addictive drugs can serve as reinforcers in conditioning experiments in much the same way as food or sex. Defined as an event that strengthens the likelihood that the preceding behaviour will recur, a reinforcer can be described as either positive or negative in action. A positive reinforcer acts by inducing a novel state and a negative reinforcer reduces an aversive state. Drugs of abuse can serve as both positive and negative reinforcers. For example, when a drug alleviates the symptoms of withdrawal it is acting as a negative reinforcer and when a drug induces a state of euphoria it is acting as a positive reinforcer.

Research in behavioural pharmacology has demonstrated that drug seeking behaviour is maintained by many of the same learning processes that are thought to influence behaviour maintained by non-drug rewards. One important finding is that environmental stimuli associated with drug taking such as drug paraphernalia can come to exert conditioned effects in their own right and that such effects may be involved in the phenomena of drug craving (Goldberg and Stolerman, 1986).

This finding has led to the development of a novel treatment approach known as cue exposure that aims to break down the conditioned drug effects that are thought to contribute to the behavioural pattern of drug seeking that characterises an addiction (Drummond *et al.*, 1995).

Cue exposure is based on the principle of classical (also called Pavlovian) extinction. At its most basic level cue exposure is built on the premise that repeated, non-reinforced exposure to drug cues (e.g. the sight of a syringe) will diminish any conditioned drug effects. Since these conditioned drug effects are thought to be closely related to the notions of craving and relapse, it follows that cue exposure holds some promise as a component treatment for drug addiction. Indeed, there is some evidence to suggest that cue exposure can provide a useful adjunct to therapy (O'Brien and Childress, 1991). It is also been demonstrated that exposing cocaine dependent outpatients to cocaine-related stimuli did not increase the risk of subsequent drug taking (Ehrman *et al.*, 1998). However, it is generally agreed that the utility of this approach as a behavioural intervention in outpatient settings remains to be seen (Dawe *et al.*, 1993).

COGNITIVE THEORIES

"There are sores which slowly erode the mind in solitude like a kind of canker... relief is to be found only in the oblivion brought about by wine and in the artificial sleep induced by opium and similar narcotics. Alas, the effects of such medicines are only temporary. After a certain point, instead of alleviating the pain they only intensify it" (Sadegh Hedyat, 1997, p. 1).

Undoubtedly behavioural pharmacology has made a significant contribution to our understanding of the conditioning and learning processes involved in the development of drug addiction. However, behavioural theorists have been criticised for failing to acknowledge that human drug use is influenced by social and economic factors, as well as previously acquired expectancies and/or belief systems about drugs. In contrast the focus of the cognitive approach is on cognitive states, with treatment being directed towards changing what are thought to be unhelpful belief systems that can lead to continued drug use or relapse.

The idea that individuals will use drugs to change their internal cognitive states is by no means new. Some forms of religious experience can be attributed to drug use, as can many creative and artistic accomplishments. However, while drugs can be used as a means of enhancing everyday and creative functioning they are more likely to be used as a means of minimising unpleasant thoughts and beliefs about the self. The Regulation of Cognitive States (RCS) model (Toneatto, 1995) is a promising model based on this idea. This model argues that the compulsive drug seeking behaviour is maintained over time because the drug effect induces a change in perceptions, thoughts, sensations, memories, imagery and/or emotions from a less preferred to a more preferred state. Treatment thus aims to help clients identify those cognitive states that are regularly avoided through the use of substances. Toneatto suggests that treatment congruent with the RCS model should help clients to become more aware of their cognitive states and learn to regulate uncomfortable states of awareness without modifying them pharmacologically.

COGNITIVE-BEHAVIOURAL THEORIES

"But don't tell me you can't kick it if you want to. When I hear a junkie tell me he wants to kick the habit but he just can't I know he lies even if he don't know he does." (Nelson Algren, 1998, p. 63).

With its roots in social-learning theory (Bandura, 1977), the third approach to addiction views the compulsive drug seeking behaviour thought to characterise an addiction as overlearned, maladaptive habit patterns. Based on this model, relapse prevention is a treatment approach which places addiction on a continuum with normal drug taking behaviour and acknowledges the important role that situational and environmental factors play in the development and maintenance of addiction. The use of this treatment approach in both inpatient and outpatient treatment settings has been demonstrated by Marlatt and his colleagues (e.g. Marlatt and Gordon, 1985). Essentially this is a cognitive-behavioural self-management treatment programme focussing on the identification of high-risk situations, cues, triggers and other factors that may lead to relapse.

The general aims of relapse prevention are to provide the individual with the skills to avoid lapses, to prevent lapses from becoming relapses and to reduce the negative consequences of relapse (Andrews and Jenkins, 1999). These goals are achieved by forming a working relationship and therapeutic alliance with clients and undertaking appropriate prevention strategies such as promoting the client's insight and awareness, promoting skills and behavioural repertoires of action, challenging unhelpful beliefs and promoting healthy lifestyle changes.

There are a number of key elements to relapse prevention. Of particular importance is establishing a clear understanding between the client and the professional as to the role that relapse prevention plays in the decision to change behaviour. Although relapse prevention tends to be thought of as a strategy to adopt when in the maintenance stage of change, its use is in fact much broader than this. Thus, within a harm minimisation model of therapy in which abstinence is not the agreed goal, the avoidance of previous risky behaviours may be seen as an important part of the relapse prevention process.

It is argued that having a balanced lifestyle is central to the avoidance of relapse. The desire for "indulgence" through the use of substances is seen as a form of lifestyle imbalance and one that leads to potential high-risk situations. For the client any change in behaviour towards their substance misuse can lead to urges or cravings, particularly where a positive outcome is anticipated. Even where such urges or cravings are not being experienced, clients may find that they place themselves in high-risk situations with seeming abandon. Thus, within the cognitive-behavioural model of relapse it is argued that clients may take what are called "seemingly irrelevant decisions" in which they are at high risk of lapsing. An example of a "seemingly irrelevant decision" would be the individual, who has stopped using, going for a drink in the pub their dealer frequents. A high-risk situation is thus established, although from the individual's perspective there may be a denial of any intentionality: after all they just wanted a drink and it just so happened that they chose their dealer's pub!

When clients do find themselves in such high-risk situations their coping strategies come into play. With good coping strategies the client will increase their self-efficacy and thereby reduce their risk of relapse. On the other hand, where there are poor coping strategies and a belief in a positive outcome from the addictive behaviour, a slip or lapse is increasingly likely.

If a lapse does occur it is important that all or nothing is avoided, so that clients do not think that a lapse signals or predicts a full-blown relapse. Of particular importance in this regard is what is known as the rule-violation effect. Where clients establish a rule for themselves, e.g. abstinence, substance reduction, avoidance of high-risk behaviour, they can, if a slip takes place, believe that a relapse is inevitable as essentially they are unable to reconcile their action with their aspirations. Where lapses do occur, they should be used to learn and bolster coping strategies rather than simply being interpreted as a sign of failure. It is also a useful opportunity to reflect upon lifestyle balance and to remind clients of the positive changes that they made prior to such lapses occurring.

Wanigaratne (2000) has usefully constructed a ten-point checklist for therapists in order to ensure that they are operating relapse prevention strategies at their optimum level:

A TEN-POINT CHECKLIST FOR RELAPSE PREVENTION THERAPISTS

1. Identification of high-risk situations and classically conditioned cues (triggers) for craving.
2. Initial development of strategies to limit exposure to high-risk situations.
3. Development of skills to successfully endure cravings and other painful effects.
4. Development of skills to deal with other high-risk situations that could be peculiar to the individual.
5. Learning to cope with lapses.
6. Learning how to challenge and or better manage maladaptive thoughts about substance use.
7. Learning how to avoid using when one is in an otherwise unavoidable high-risk situation.
8. Generating a basic emergency plan for coping with a high-risk situation when other skills are not working.
9. Learning to detect various ways in which one is "setting oneself up" to use substances.
10. Generating pleasurable sober activities and relationships to offset feelings of emptiness and loss after removal of substance use.

Whilst the provision of relapse prevention therapy requires a trained practitioner, the above list provides a useful starting point from which community pharmacists can engage clients in conversations about their drug use.

STAGES OF CHANGE MODEL
The phenomenon of motivation is central to our understanding of addiction (Miller, 1996). Research and theory have linked the concept of motivation to our understanding of how an addiction can develop and how an addiction can seem to disappear. How do some people escape from the compulsive pattern of drug seeking that once overwhelmed their existence? A useful theoretical model that provides some insight to the answer of this question is the Stages of Change Model (Prochaska and DiClemente, 1986), and is one with which many pharmacists engaged in health promotion will be familiar. Developed from work with problem drinkers, this empirically derived model is widely used to help explain the fundamental role that motivation plays in changing an addictive behaviour. One of the most important findings that has come from research using this model of change, is that enduring behaviour change is driven in part by the strength of commitment to change in the first place. In order to escape from addiction there must be a strong commitment to change. In fact, in order for someone to benefit from any psychological intervention for drug addiction there must be a strong commitment to change.

Using the Stages of Change Model (see Figure 15.1), it is possible to track how ready someone is to benefit from treatment. The first stage of this model describes the stage of motivation when drug users are yet to contemplate changing their behaviour. This stage is known as the Precontemplation stage. Once an individual begins

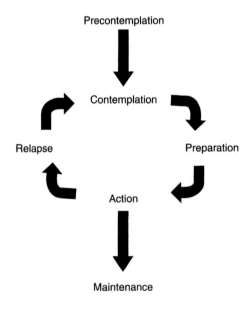

Figure 15.1 The stages of change model.

to consider the possibility of change, he or she is said to enter the next stage known as the Contemplation stage and may apply, in a pharmacy context, to needle exchange clients who are not actively seeking treatment. The model suggests that although an individual in the Contemplation stage is considering change, their ability to do so is likely to be immobilised. It is not until someone reaches the Action stage when overt attempts to change first occur and the individual is then ready to benefit from psychological intervention designed to maintain a change in addictive behaviour over time. Patients on a methadone prescription will have been in the Action phase with regard to treatment-seeking. However, they may only be in the Contemplation phase with regard to intermediate goals, such as moving from injecting illicit drugs used in addition to their prescribed methadone, to using them orally, abstaining from illicit drug use completely, to the ultimate goal of becoming drug-free entirely.

MOTIVATIONAL INTERVIEWING

As mentioned already, it has been demonstrated that psychological intervention aimed at maintaining change in addictive behaviour will not be effective unless the individual receiving the intervention is in the Action stage of changing behaviour. However, that is not to say that there is nothing that a drug worker or pharmacist can achieve with a client who has not yet reached the Action stage. Using a client-centred counselling style that aims to work with ambivalence and effectively mobilise an individual's ability to change, there is growing acknowledgement that drug-workers can guide a client from the Contemplation stage towards the Action stage of change. Termed Motivational Interviewing (MI), this counselling style has been shown to be a useful precursor to psychological intervention packages for addiction as well as other behaviours such as offending (Miller and Rollnick, 1991). MI attempts to allow the client to develop ambivalence around their drug use. In its most simple level this may involve asking the client to describe what is good about their drug use and then to describe what is not so good, without the "counsellor" being directive or instructing someone on the best course of action by which to solve any problems. Research into the use of "MI-style" techniques in a community pharmacy context is currently underway in the areas of smoking cessation and misuse of over-the-counter analgesics and preliminary results look promising.

Rollnick and Miller describe a number of characteristics of MI:

- "Motivation to change is elicited from the client, and not imposed from without".
- "It is the client's task, not the counsellor's, to articulate and resolve his or her ambivalence, ... for example, 'If I stop smoking I will feel better about myself, but I may also put on weight, which will make me feel unhappy and unattractive'". The counsellor then guides the client towards an acceptable solution.
- "Direct persuasion is not an effective method for resolving ambivalence". However tempting, the counsellor should not "help" the client by trying to get them to see that they need to change urgently.
- "The counselling style is generally a quiet and eliciting one".
- "The counsellor is directive in helping the client to examine and resolve ambivalence".

- "Readiness to change is not a client trait, but a fluctuating product of interpersonal interaction".
- "The therapeutic relationship is more like a partnership or companionship than expert/recipient roles" (Rollnick and Miller, 1995).

There are a growing number of research studies that claim that Motivational Interviewing offers a very useful psychological intervention that can serve as a pre-cursor to treatment (Saunders, Wilkinson and Phillips, 1995). Once an individual is ready to change and is ready for treatment it is then appropriate to conduct a thor-ough psychological assessment in order to match that individual to the psychological intervention for addiction that is suited best to their needs (Project Match Research Group, 1997).

BRIEF INTERVENTIONS

Though not strictly speaking based on psychological theories, brief interventions form an important part of the "talking therapies" response to drug misuse, in particular with regard to stimulating behaviour change. A brief intervention has the following characteristics:

- Time limited to 5–10 minutes.
- Patient-centred counselling strategy.
- Focus on behaviour change.
- Increased compliance with desired behaviours.
- Followed up (adapted from Fleming and Manwell, 1999).

It has been shown that GPs who deliver opportunistic brief interventions with patients have been able to get them to reduce their alcohol intake (Heather, 1995). Like their GP colleagues, community pharmacists are ideally placed to deliver brief interven-tions, around areas such as the safe storage of take-home methadone, or vaccination for hepatitis B. The development and testing of such interventions in collaboration with specialists in the field could provide pharmacists with a new set of tools for deliv-ering health promotion messages.

CONCLUSION

This chapter has introduced the reader to a number of theories of addiction, as well as some of the therapeutic applications arising from such theories. Three theories in particular, behavioural, cognitive and cognitive-behavioural have been described more fully. Some of the treatments arising from these theories as well as some of the research evidence have been outlined. Perhaps the most useful treatment interven-tions for those working in community settings are the ideas found within motivational interviewing and relapse prevention programmes and it is not unreasonable to expect that community pharmacists trained in these techniques could have a positive impact on the health and welfare of their patients. The question of how such techniques can be utilised in practice remains open, and yet to be determined. Furthermore, the skilled application of these techniques requires more than just exposure to the written word. The techniques described above can be seen as a useful starting point, allowing the opportunity for more systematic development and implementation.

REFERENCES

Algren N (1998). *The Man with the Golden Arm*. Rebel Inc, Edinburgh.

Anderson C, Blenkinsopp A (2001). Health, Disease and Health Education. In Harman RJ (ed). *Handbook of pharmacy health education* (2nd edition), Pharmaceutical Press, London.

Andrews G, Jenkins R (1999). Substance Use Disorders. In Andrews G, Jenkins R (eds). *Management of Mental Disorders*, World Health Organization Collaborating Centres in Mental Health, Sydney and London.

Ball JC, Ross A (1991). *The Effectiveness of Methadone Maintenance Treatment: Patients, Programmes, Services, and Outcome*, New York: Springer-Verlag.

Bandura A (1977). *Social Learning Theory*, Prentice-Hall, Englewood Cliffs NJ.

Burroughs W (1977). *Junky*, Penguin, Harmondsworth.

Dawe S, Powell J, Richards D, Gossop M, Marks I, Strang J, Gray JA (1993). Does post-withdrawal cue exposure improve outcome in opiate addiction? A controlled trial. *Addiction*, 88, 1233–1245.

Drummond DC, Tiffany ST, Glautier SP, Remington B (Eds.) (1995). *Addictive Behaviour: Cue Exposure Theory and Practice*, John Wiley, Chichester.

Ehrman RN, Robbins SJ, Childress AR, Goehl L, Hole AV, O'Brian CP (1998). Laboratory exposure to cocaine cues does not increase cocaine use by outpatient subjects. *Journal of Substance Abuse Treatment*, 15, 431–435.

Fleming M, Manwell LB (1999). Brief intervention in primary care settings. A primary treatment method for at-risk, problem, and dependent drinkers. *Alcohol Research and Health*. 23, 128–37.

Goldberg SR, Stolerman IP (Eds.) (1986). *Behavioral Analysis of Drug Dependence*, Academic Press, New York.

Heather N (1995). Interpreting the evidence on brief interventions for excessive drinkers: the need for caution. *Alcohol and Alcoholism*, 30, 287–296.

Hedyat S (1997). *The Blind Owl*, Rebel Press, Edinburgh.

Jaffe J (1975). Drug Addiction and Drug Abuse. In Goddman LS, Filman A (Eds.). *The Pharmacological Bases of Therapeutics*, Macmillan, New York.

Kavan A (1970). High in the Mountains. In *Julia and the Bazooka*, New York, Norton.

Marlatt GA, Gordon JR (1985). *Relapse Prevention: Maintenance strategies in the treatment of addictive behaviours*, Guilford Press, New York.

Mattick R, Ward J, Hall W (1998). The Role of Counselling and Psychological Therapy. In Ward J, Mattick RP, Hall W (Eds.). *Methadone Maintenance Treatment and Other Opioid Replacement Therapies*, Harwood Academic, Australia.

Miller WR, Rollnick S (1991). *Motivational Interviewing: Preparing people to change addictive behaviour*, Guilford Press, New York.

Miller WR (1996). Motivational interviewing: Research, practice and puzzles. *Addictive Behaviours*, 61, 835–842.

O'Brien C, Childress AR (1991). Behaviour Therapy for Drug Dependence. In Glass I (Ed.) *The International Handbook of Addiction Behaviour*, Routledge, London.

Orford J (2001). Addiction as excessive appetite. *Addiction*, 96, 1, 15–33.

Prochaska JO, DiClemente CC (1986). Toward a Comprehensive Model of Change. In Miller WR and Heather N (Eds.). *Treating Addictive Behaviours: Processes of change*, Plenum, New York.

Project Match Research Group (1997). Matching alcoholism treatments to client's heterogeneity: project MATCH post-treatment drinking outcomes. *Journal of Studies in Alcohol*, 58, 7–29.

Rollnick S, Miller WR (1995). What is MI? *Behavioural and Cognitive Psychotherapy*, 23, 325–334.

Saunders B, Wilkinson C, Phillips M (1995). The impact of brief motivational intervention with opiate users attending a methadone programme. *Addiction*, 90, 3, 415–424.

Sinclair HK, Bond CM, Lennox AS, *et al.* (1995). Nicotine replacement therapies: smoking cessation outcomes in a pharmacy setting in Scotland. *Tobacco Control*, 4, 338–343.

Toneatto T (1995). The regulation of cognitive states: A cognitive model of psychoactive substance abuse. *Journal of Cognitive Psychotherapy: An International Quarterly*, 9, 93–103.

Wanigaratne S (2000). *A Ten-Point Checklist for Relapse Prevention Therapists.* Internal Psychology Document, South London and Maudsley NHS Trust, London.

Wertz JM, Sayette MA (2001). A review of the effects of perceived drug use opportunity on self-reported urge. *Experimental and Clinical Psychopharmacology*, 9, 3–13.

West R (2001). Theories of addiction. *Addiction*, 96, 3–15.

16

Shared care at the primary and secondary interface: GPs and specialist drug services

Emily Finch and Chris Ford

This chapter describes the background to the current focus on the shared care of drug users in the UK, describing the roles of primary and secondary (specialist) health care providers, and the way in which community pharmacy interfaces with them in respect of the care and treatment of drug users.

BACKGROUND

The treatment of drug misuse varies from country to country, but in general, the availability of treatment and recommended practice are influenced by committees, advisory bodies and government guidelines. In the UK, the system is more flexible and less regulated, and has allowed emergence of an approach described as the "British System". This is covered in more detail in Chapter 2.

The UK has an extraordinary network of more than 35,000 general practitioners (GPs), providing primary health care to a locally defined population, with about 97% of the population registered with a GP. Up until the mid-1960s, treatment for the extremely small number of opiate addicts being provided by GPs was for either gradual withdrawal or, if attempts to stop failed and the patient could function well with a regular supply, then maintenance was acceptable. Such treatment gradually became an acceptable part of service provision. These addict patients were middle-aged or elderly, and many were either "therapeutic addicts" (i.e. had become addicted through the use of opiates for therapeutic purposes) or "professional addicts" (e.g. doctors). There was no "system" of treatment or legal dose limits, but as the number of addicts was small this was not considered important.

In the 1960s, a new group of young heroin users emerged who used prescribed drugs obtained from the illicit market for recreational purposes. The 1965 Brain Committee concluded that the increase in drug use was mostly the result of over-prescribing by doctors leading to the diversion of prescriptions onto the illicit market (HMSO, 1965). It was therefore recommended that the management of these addicts should be taken over by psychiatrists instead of GPs, reversing the recommendations of the original Brain Committee (see Chapters 2 and 3).

There was also a recommendation to establish new specialist drug treatment centres. These new drug dependency units (DDU) or clinics were set up in 1968 (mainly in London). Initially the clinics prescribed heroin, then oral and injectable methadone (Mitcheson, 1994). No one foresaw the extent to which drug misuse was to increase because of increased availability and the introduction of smokable heroin. As the number of people seeking treatment continued to grow and these specialist services became overwhelmed, the clinic staff tired of their accumulating caseloads and their clients continued drug use and injecting behaviours, and they began to question the benefits of maintenance and injectable prescribing (Strang, 1984). The subsequent debate about the different dosage forms of opiate prescribing – reinforced by an inconclusive study comparing injectable heroin maintenance to oral methadone (Hartnoll *et al.*, 1980) – resulted in most clinics moving to oral methadone by the end of the 1970s.

The clinics were also instructed by the Ministry of Health to encourage eventual withdrawal and prescribe minimum quantities to reduce the threat of diversion. By the early 1980s many of the clinics had moved from maintenance to detoxification regimens. This was also the time that GPs were again asked to play a role in this area of work when in 1982 the ACMD (Advisory Council on the Misuse of Drugs) were concerned about the increasing and varying drug problem. They recommended a possible role for some doctors outside the specialist services, with safeguards (Department of Health and Social Security, 1982). This was followed by the publication by the Department of Health, of Guidelines for doctors – guidance which was endorsed by the British Medical Association and the negotiating body for general practice, the GMSC (Department of Health and Social Security, 1984). This was taken up by some GPs (Glanz and Taylor, 1986), although their individual involvement remained low (Tantam *et al.*, 1993). Community Drug Teams (CDTs) were also established to support GPs in the active treatment of drug problems (Strang *et al.*, 1992; Strang and Clements, 1994) (see below).

By the mid-1980s, the goals for drug treatment had changed again. Accompanying a continued rise in drug use, a growing public awareness of a potential HIV epidemic, and the failure of abstinence treatment, there was a move back towards maintenance prescribing with harm reduction as the new treatment goal. The 1988 ACMD report was important and led to a change in how many drug services worked with their clients. It stated that HIV was a greater threat to individual and public health than drug use *per se*. Outreach services and needle exchanges were introduced. Because of the need to increase the prescribing base, GPs were seen to have a key role in limiting the spread of HIV amongst drug users. Harm reduction was embraced as a general objective by the majority of services, but there was uncertainty as to whether maintenance prescribing was, or was not, the most effective way of achieving harm reduction. Thus, needle exchange schemes were generally supported, whilst different prescribing options were the subject of more uncertainty. This left many drug users outside the system and their only choices were private prescribers or the few NHS GPs who were willing to care for these patients and prescribe maintenance.

These GPs were usually very committed to this area of work and saw the benefits in their patients of stabilisation of lifestyle, improvement in health and reduction in the need for their patients to turn to crime to fund their drug habit. The GPs who did get involved were rarely supported and tended to attract larger numbers of drug users than perhaps could be easily managed in one general practice.

In 1995 as a result of *Tackling Drugs Together* (HMSO, 1995) there was a NHS Executive letter sent to all health authorities asking them to review their "Shared Care Arrangements for Drug Users" (NHS Executive, 1995). Only 26 of the 120 health authorities had shared care arrangements in place, with the content of these differing widely (Gerada and Tighe, 1999). Over the next few years, health authorities increased their shared care provision, although there is still substantial variation in the type of model of care provided.

Community drug teams and drug dependence units continue to provide care for drug users although the services they provide have developed since their inception. These are also described below.

CURRENT STRUCTURE OF DRUG SERVICES
(a) Role of the GP
To date, there is a wide variation in GP involvement with drug users. Many GPs are committed to working with drug users whereas others do not want to prescribe for them. One survey found that 18% of GPs were undertaking total care of some drug users and that 47% would take on prescribing if requested by a specialist or as part of a joint care programme (Pirie and Ryan, 1999), whilst another study, broadly con-temporary, found that GPs were generally unwilling to work with drug users (Deehan *et al.*, 1997). Other studies showed that with the right support and training GPs were willing to undertake this area of work (Ryrie *et al.*, 1999). In the 1995 national survey of community pharmacies, 40% of the prescriptions dispensed by community phar-macists, for drug users, were written by GPs (Strang *et al.*, 1996). Both the 1999 Departments of Health guidelines and the preceding 1991 guidelines state that the general health problems of drug users should be treated by GPs in the same way as any other patient (Departments of Health, 1999). Therefore in most cases GPs should be prepared to provide general medical care for drug users even if they do not want to prescribe substitute medication (e.g. methadone) for them. To do otherwise has been described as unacceptable and as "discrimination on the grounds of diagnosis" (Strang, 1989).

Many GPs prescribe methadone either as part of a reduction programme or for maintenance. Indeed methadone maintenance may be particularly suitable for prescribing in general practice. Some GPs only see one or two drug users in the context of a general practice list but others, who have been called "specialised generalists" (Departments of Health, 1999), may provide total care to many more drug users. These GPs may deliver a fuller range of prescribing options. GPs may, either alone or in the context of a shared care scheme (see below), provide drug counselling, harm reduction advice and specialist medical care such as HIV and hepatitis testing and hepatitis B vaccination, as well as the normal full primary health care.

GP prescribing has many advantages. GPs tend to be more flexible, they do not have waiting lists and can often respond quickly to a patient's needs. They can pro-vide the range of medical care, such as contraception and antenatal care in conjunc-tion with substitute prescribing, leading to a more holistic package of care.

However most GPs have had no training in drug dependency, and hence lack the confidence and the skills needed to manage drug users. Some may perceive drug users as being difficult individuals, particularly if they have had no support and training. Training for GPs should be an integral part of shared care schemes, but sadly this is not always the case. Where it has been an integral part of the scheme and provided by primary care specialists, it has been found to be effective (Ford and Ryrie, 2000). More training is needed at undergraduate and post-graduate level, with curricula being modified to incorporate this field. There could also special courses for GPs who wish to become more specialised in managing drug users.

The Department of Health has now recognised the importance of training. Since 2001 there have been three new training initiatives in England and Wales, with others being developed in Scotland. In England a certificate course is being developed for GPs who are already doing this work, or who wish to become more specialised and need consolidation of their clinical skills. In conjunction with an academic unit, a diploma course is also being developed which will look at the wider aspects of managing drug misuse. A third initiative is providing basic awareness training for GPs, hospital doctors and other primary health professionals.

(b) Community drug teams

Since the late 1980s methadone treatment in the UK has largely been delivered by Community Drug Teams (CDTs). Their structure and function has been reviewed by Strang *et al.* (1992). They were first suggested as a way of organising treatment delivery to drug users by the *Treatment and Rehabilitation Report* from the Advisory Council on the Misuse of Drugs (ACMD) published in 1982. Using community teams to provide services for drug users was a concept borrowed from community alcohol and community mental handicap teams (Clement, 1989). By the mid-1980s they were being set up rapidly, following the central funding initiative which was given £17 million to implement the scheme (MacGregor *et al.*, 1990).

Between 1984 and 1988, 62 community drug teams were established. It was conceived that the CDTs would take on the GPs as their "clients" and the GPs would be able to take on a larger number of drug users. However, it was precisely in this area that their impact was found to be lacking and despite being popular and broadly welcomed, their introduction was actually associated with a reduction in GP caseload, as the new community drug teams took on the GPs' caseload rather than the GPs themselves.

All areas of the UK now have some form of community drug service. Funding and management vary substantially with some services being run by non-statutory organisations and others by local NHS trusts. Both their structure and function vary substantially across the UK (Strang *et al.*, 1992).

A study carried out in 1991 found that the average CDT is staffed by a mixture of full- and part-time workers – usually two community psychiatric nurses, one social worker, a secretary and a co-ordinator (Strang *et al.*, 1992) although many also employ drug workers and psychologists.

The function of CDTs also varies. Some provide advice and counselling only (often including needle exchange), but more have some type of prescribing service. They may either employ a local GP for a number of sessions or have a relationship with local GPs and manage patients using a shared care model. Some services have medical staff working in the team – either clinical assistants, local GPs with a special interest or consultant psychiatrists. Opiate dependency is usually the focus of treatment, and some have fallen short of addressing increasing polydrug use, concurrent alcohol use or other primary drug problems.

Within a community drug team, workers have a caseload of patients whom they see regularly. An opiate user on a methadone prescription will have a keyworker who manages their care, including making many decisions about their methadone prescription, although the final responsibility for the prescription does, of course, rest with the doctor.

Through the late 1990s, in many geographical areas there was increasingly an attempt to provide integrated drug services, with social care teams who fund rehabilitation care packages working in close partnership with community drug teams. In some areas the teams are now fully integrated.

(c) DDUs

As described earlier, the Drug Dependence Units were set up between 1968 and 1970. They only served small areas of they country and were mostly set up in London. They have changed substantially since then and most have some form of community drug service attached to them. The boundary between a community drug team and a drug dependency unit may be blurred in some areas.

DDUs are attached to local mental health services and are typically headed by a consultant psychiatrist who is usually a specialist in substance misuse. Many DDUs provide services for drug (mostly opiate) users and alcohol users. DDUs are staffed similarly to community drug teams, with nurses and drug workers keyworking clients, although there may be more medical input with junior medical staff also having caseloads of clients. A DDU may also provide training for nurses and medical staff.

DDUs may provide a range of prescribing options. They may provide specialist prescribing options such as injectable medication, although there is a substantial national variation in the amount of these options available. Traditionally they provide care for opiate users only and are now having to respond to the treatment needs of stimulant users and polydrug users. They may, in partnership with mental health services, provide care for clients who have co-morbidity (concurrent mental health and substance misuse) problems.

Some DDUs have inpatient units with facilities to provide detoxification and stabilisation. Increasingly, however, inpatient detoxification services are provided for an area by services outside the geographical area, possibly even in the private sector. Some areas have a few beds within a local psychiatric facility only, despite evidence that inpatient detoxification is more successful in specialist units (Strang *et al.*, 1997). As with community drug teams, in some areas social service care managers may also be co-located with a DDU.

INTEGRATING THE THERAPEUTIC ACTIVITIES – SHARED CARE

Shared care is the joint participation of GPs and specialists (and others as appropriate) in the planned delivery of care for patients with a drug misuse problem (Department of Health, 1996). It is now an integral component of Britain's drug policy (HMSO, 1995) and treatment guidelines (Departments of Health, 1999). The term "shared care" is open to numerous interpretations. This is a complex term and often poorly defined. In drug service terms it is used to mean the sharing of responsibility for providing care for drug users and sharing of information about their care, between primary care (GP) and the secondary services (specialists).

The UK Clinical Guidelines define "shared care" as the joint participation of GPs and specialists (CDTs, DDUs and other agencies as appropriate) in the planned delivery of care for patients with a drug misuse problem, informed by an enhanced information exchange beyond routine discharge and referral letter (Departments of Health, 1999). No single ideal model of shared care suits all areas, and models need to be developed around local history and service provision. Examples include the scheme in Glasgow where all prescribing is done by GPs who are supported by counsellors from a community drug team (Gruer *et al.*, 1997). Schemes in Edinburgh (Greenwood, 1990) and Brent and Harrow (North London) (Ryrie *et al.*, 1999) and South London (Groves *et al.*, 2000) have a dedicated team who support and train GPs to work with drug users. The user is encouraged to register with a GP and is then referred to the specialist team for initial prescribing and stabilisation. The stable drug user is then referred back to the GP for ongoing prescribing (Bury, 1995). There are a growing number of shared care services which are primary care led, the biggest of these is the Wirral Drug Services.

In other areas, drug users are assessed by specialist services and prescribed for by their GP with daily supervised dispensing by community pharmacists, while maintaining regular contact with specialist services for further counselling and support. Some areas use a four-way agreement between the client, GP, specialist service and dispensing pharmacy which provides a format in which all parties are aware of service requirements and this facilitates communication (Walker, 2001). However, there are many areas where GPs are treating drug users, with no drug specialist support as there is often no specialist service or the specialist service is unsure of how to work with primary care. In these areas, the community pharmacy may be the only source of support.

It is important to consider the local history of service provision before choosing a particular strategic approach (Barnard and Higson, 1999). For instance it may be easier to involve GPs when there has been no history of central prescribing or when shared care was an integral element from the beginning so local GPs had not seen the work as someone else's. Shared care schemes tagged onto established drug services without any changes in power or resources on the whole do not affect the number of drug users being seen in primary care. Some successful shared care schemes have been led by local GPs and may have resulted in a major overhaul of the local specialist services (Ryrie *et al.*, 1999). Successful schemes have also taken on training and supporting GPs to work with drug users.

Good practice for treatment for drug users
(i) Prescribing
All doctors in the UK can prescribe methadone for opiate addicts in any dosage form (oral mixture, tablet or ampoules). Indeed, there are no legal restrictions on what a doctor can prescribe, apart from heroin (diamorphine), cocaine and dipipanone (Diconal). For these the doctor must have a licence from the Home Office, if the drug is to be prescribed for the treatment of drug dependence, and in practice these licences are only issued to drug addiction specialists. Currently, the UK Home Office is reviewing the licencing system, which may be extended to many more controlled drugs, with the exception of methadone mixture.

The vast variation in the structure and functions of drug services in the UK makes it difficult for pharmacists to know what standards of care to expect for drug users from doctors. Indeed there are some services, long-term or maintenance prescribing for instance, which in some parts of the country are provided as standard, but which are hardly available in other areas. Provision for supervised consumption of methadone in pharmacies or in methadone clinics is available in some areas, but not in others.

In 1984, and again in 1991 and 1999, the Department of Health (Department of Health and Social Security, 1984; Departments of Health, 1991, 1999) produced guidelines for the treatment of drug dependency. The Guidelines were aimed mainly at doctors. As the 1991 Guidelines made clear, they had been prepared primarily "by doctors, for doctors", although of course utilising the joint working relationships with which the doctor was involved. These guidelines set out the opinions on best practice of a group of medical experts in the field. The 1999 Guidelines represent a gold standard of practice in prescribing for drug users and they have generally been welcomed, although they have been criticised for being too inflexible (*Druglink*, 1999). While not legally binding, those prescribing in a way which is outside the recommendations in the Guidelines may now be required to defend their prescribing. Also the evidence base for most treatments for drug misuse is very limited, which has made it difficult to describe protocols and ways of working which are supported by research evidence. This could make it difficult to prescribe treatments that have not been evidence tested, such as the use of dihydrocodeine rather than methadone in non-injectors. Some of the content of the Guidelines have serious cost implications – such as the wider provision of long-term treatment and universal provision of supervised methadone at the beginning of a treatment episode.

The Guidelines provide guidance for the prescriber about the management of drug dependence including suggested dose reduction regimes, protocols for dose stabilisation and supervision of methadone consumption, the improvement of compliance and the management of clients on methadone maintenance.

The Guidelines also describe the role of the community pharmacist and recommend that GPs and drug workers liaise with them when prescribing. This aspect is considered more fully later in this chapter, as well as elsewhere within this book. Pharmacists can reasonably expect that doctors will provide care for clients which meets the standards described in the prescribing guidelines. In some areas, health commissioners may choose to ignore some recommendations, such as the provision of supervised methadone, because of cost pressures and therefore make it difficult for the doctor and/or the pharmacist to provide this.

(ii) Ethics

Harm reduction involves accepting that a drug user may continue to take drugs, but that the intervention or treatment he or she receives will reduce the harm either to the individual or to society. For instance, when one dependence-forming drug (usually heroin) is replaced by another dependence-forming drug (usually methadone) a prescriber must establish that the individual is benefiting despite his continued dependence. Evidence would suggest that clients usually do benefit from treatment (Department of Health, 1996). A doctor also has an ethical obligation to prescribe drugs responsibly to bring about a health benefit for their patient and accept appropriate peer support and guidance.

Some doctors, as discussed earlier, refuse to manage drug users and some even refuse to care for drug users' general medical problems. The General Medical Council (GMC) states that: "it is ... unethical for a doctor to withhold treatment from any patient on the basis of a moral judgement that the patient's activities or lifestyle might have contributed to the condition for which treatment is being sought" (Departments of Health, 1999) and doctors should not allow their own views or prejudices to cloud their clinical judgements. In some ways there are parallels here for the pharmacy profession; many community pharmacists refuse to dispense to drug users, often due to moral judgements about drug misuse. Again, such judgements have no place in deciding whether or not to provide services.

Patient confidentiality is an essential requirement for the preservation of trust between patients and all health professionals. A clear consistent approach is necessary. A team that includes the GP, the drug worker and the pharmacist should be clear about which types of information can and need to be shared. Information about drug users should only be released to other outside agencies when the individual has given clear consent.

Drug users present dilemmas about confidentiality. They may often be engaged in illegal activities and, in order to maintain a productive therapeutic relationship with a client, professionals usually decide not disclose these activities to the police. The incident in 1999, when two professionals working for the "Wintercomfort" agency in Cambridge were jailed for failing to report drug dealing to the police, has made drug agencies revisit their confidentiality policies (Shapiro, 2000). Very rarely this confidentiality may be breached. Confidentiality can also be breached when a child is at risk of serious harm.

The treatment of young people under the age of 16 presents particular ethical issues especially with regard to needle exchange and prescribing. In general, any intervention for a young person is best provided with the consent of their parents or guardian. If the young person does not want their parents to know, the intervention can still be provided unless there are clear contraindications for doing so. The Standing Conference on Drug Abuse (SCODA) have produced guidelines on the treatment of young people and drug action teams may have local ones (Dale-Perera *et al.*, 1999).

In most patient–prescriber relationships the patient has a clear right to information about their treatment and to make choices about their prescription depending on that information. When a doctor is prescribing substitute medication (such as methadone) for an opiate user, however, the doctor's judgement and the patient's choices may differ. Given the patient's addiction, their choice of drug may be in danger of being influenced excessively by the intoxicant potential of the drug, rather than its ability to confer actual health gain, for example. A patient may want a higher dose of medication to provide a euphoriant effect and a doctor may only want to prescribe to relieve the symptoms of withdrawal. Whenever possible, in these circumstances, doctors need to satisfy themselves that their clinical decision is the correct one for the patient which will produce optimal outcome. Whenever possible the prescribing doctor and client should come to a joint decision.

Unlike many conditions, drug misuse affects both the individual and wider society. For instance the benefits of treatment may be those which affect society, such as reduction in criminal activity. The disadvantages of treatment, such as the diversion of methadone onto the illicit drug market, may have adverse effects on other individuals if the methadone is taken illicitly or accidentally, possibly leading to overdose deaths (Binchy *et al.*, 1994; Roberts *et al.*, 1997).

The treatment offered to an individual drug user may affect the treatment expectations of others. Even though the doctor and other health care personnel may be bound by confidentiality, the patient is not constrained in this way. Some patients may readily divulge, or even brag about, the specific drug, the dose or the dispensing arrangements. A doctor who prescribes diamorphine or other injectable opiates for drug users may inadvertently raise expectations that other service users should be prescribed the same drug or the same dose. A doctor with minimal prior experience or training in this field, or little support, may be particularly at risk of being manipulated. (Similarly, inexperienced pharmacists are also at risk of being manipulated into "bending the rules".) For these reasons, the prescriber has a responsibility also to consider the potential effect of their decisions on society and on the drug misusing community.

(iii) Other treatment elements
Any treatment for a drug misuser, whether it involves prescribing or not, must have an objective and some mechanism to assess whether or not that objective has been reached. The objectives can be across a range of outcome domains, e.g. reduced illicit drug use, improved physical and mental health, improved social functioning or reduced criminal activity. For many clients improvements may initially be small, e.g. reduction in criminal activity and therefore difficult for an external observer to understand. Most patients do improve in treatment and the reduction of morbidity and mortality is enormous (ACMD, 2000), although research evidence would indicate that there is still a minority who do not (Gossop *et al.*, 1998).

A treatment package should include education about the health damage associated with illicit drug use and injecting, needle exchange, screening for HIV, hepatitis B and C, and hepatitis B vaccination should be available. Drug users should be encouraged to register with GPs. Social care needs, such as housing and benefit (welfare) advice, need to be addressed. Psychiatric care may also be needed.

Relapse prevention is the main cognitive-behavioural counselling technique used to assist drug users to reduce their drug use. Motivational interviewing has also been developed to improve treatment retention and outcome. These techniques should be available either from the prescribing doctor, or as a consequence of partnership arrangement between prescribing doctors in primary care and drug agencies.

Relationships with pharmacists
(i) Primary care/GPs
A vital cog, so easily forgotten in allowing GPs to be able to work with drug users in the community, is the community pharmacist. The pharmacist often forms a strong relationship with the drug user, whom they see more frequently than the GP, often daily. They are able to build up a picture of how the drug user is managing on treatment and can provide important information.

It is always courteous and good practice for the GP to confirm with the pharmacist, before sending a new drug misuser, that he or she is willing to dispense the prescribed drug. This can be the first step in the relationship between the pharmacist and the GP. It is useful to record the address and telephone number of the pharmacist in the GP notes and vice-versa for the pharmacist. The pharmacist should be told about any potential problems with the client, such as a concurrent alcohol problem which may result in the client attending intoxicated.

Supervised consumption can help joint working between pharmacists and pre-scribers. The pharmacist can give useful information about the patient to the pre-scriber around compliance, health and welfare of the user. The pharmacist can also help assess the suitability of a user to reduce their supervision. This can be helpful to all three parties and increases collaboration between them. Many GPs consider phar-macists to be part of the primary care team and having a named pharmacist in the notes is a key element of good management of care. Many GPs speak frequently to pharmacists about their drug-misusing patients in treatment. This contact is initiated equally by the GPs and pharmacists and valued highly by both parties.

Knowing how often prescribed medication is dispensed and the state of the drug user when he or she attends the pharmacy (e.g. whether or not they have been drink-ing or are affected by drugs) assists the doctor in assessing compliance with the treat-ment programme. The pharmacist may be able to tell the prescribing doctor about other prescribed medications dispensed, and about medication which has been bought over the counter, within the bounds of confidentiality. The pharmacist can assist in providing information about the client's general health.

(ii) Community drug teams
In most areas the community drug team has a good relationship with pharmacists who regularly dispense methadone. As with GP prescriptions, the pharmacist has a vital role in providing information on client progress.

Clients who are being treated by a community drug team typically have a key-worker who will manage their care and take a role in making decisions about their prescription in partnership with the prescriber. Therefore communication about the prescription may come from that keyworker and not from the prescriber.

As with GPs, the community drug team should check with the pharmacist by telephone or letter before a prescription is going to be presented for dispensing. It is important that they also inform the pharmacist who the keyworker is and how to make contact if there are problems with the prescription. Keyworkers should have a named pharmacist for each client and discuss any problems with them.

In many parts of the country schemes have been set up which provide super-vised administration of methadone. These schemes have improved relationships between pharmacists and community drug teams and reinforced the pharmacist's role as a member of the clinical team. Community drug teams could be involved in train-ing of pharmacists for such schemes.

(iii) DDUs
The good practice described above, such as informing pharmacists before prescrip-tions are issued, applies to DDUs as much as other treatment services. Indeed good relationships with local pharmacists may be even more important for a DDU who may have a larger number of clients, a larger proportion of whom may have addi-tional complicating problems such as co-morbid psychiatric illness, or a varying degree of liver impairment from co-morbid chronic hepatitis.

A few DDUs have their own on-site dispensing services. These will dispense methadone daily for problematic clients who are perceived as needing a maximum level of supervision and are harder to stabilise in the community. They are clients with very high need for drugs, often with co-morbidity and difficult polydrug habits. These are often staffed by specialist pharmacists, who both manage the dispensing of methadone to large numbers of clients and provide a unique resource for prescribing doctors, and more generic community pharmacists who may be managing difficult clients.

Strengthening links

Developing links between prescribing doctors and dispensing pharmacists is vital for a smooth running of any scheme caring for drug users, whether this is in specialist or primary care services. Some schemes, such as the Glasgow scheme, are dependent on GPs and pharmacists working together (Gruer *et al.*, 1997). The rise in supervised consumption has generally strengthened these relationships. These links can be developed and improved in many ways and by many forms of communication, whether it is on the phone or at meetings. Joint training sessions between pharmacists and prescribers have been found to be helpful and rewarding. The training can be on topics that are important to both, such as hepatitis B and C, HIV, new prescribing options and needle exchanges, as well as small group work looking at how to improve the local services and improve joint working.

One person who may be particularly able to help this process is the local pharmaceutical advisor or specialist pharmacist at a drug clinic, and can advise GPs and pharmacists on prescribing matters.

CONCLUSION

The interface between primary and secondary care has been changing throughout the 1990s and continues to evolve. For effective shared care, all parties involved, e.g. GPs, pharmacists and specialist services, need to be aware of each other's roles and their own strengths and weaknesses and how best to communicate with each other. As these interfaces develop and improve, so will the care of drug users.

REFERENCES

Advisory Council on the Misuse of Drugs (1988). *AIDS and Drug Misuse: Part 1*, HMSO, London.

Advisory Council on the Misuse of Drugs (2000). *Reducing Drug Related Deaths: A Report by the Advisory Council on the Misuse of Drugs*, The Stationery Office, London.

Barnard J, Higson C (1999). Caring and sharing. Modelling successful shared care. *Druglink*, January/February.

Bewley TH (1975). Evaluation of addiction treatment in England. In: Bostrom H, Larson T, Ljungsted N (eds). *Drug Dependence: Treatment and Treatment Evaluation*. Almqvist and Wiksell, Stockholm, pp. 275–286.

Binchy JM, Molyneux EM, Manning J (1994). Accidental ingestion of methadone by children in Merseyside. *British Medical Journal*, 308, 1335–1336.

Bury J (1995). Supporting GPs in Lothian to care for drug users. *International Journal of Drug Policy*, 6, 267–273.

Clement S (1989). The Community Drug Team: Lessons from Alcohol and Handicap Services. In: Bennet G (ed). *Treating Problem Drug Users*, Routledge, London.

Dale-Perera A, Hamilton C, Evans C, Britton J (1999). *Young People and Drugs: Policy Guidance for Drug Interventions*, Standing Conference on Drug Abuse. London.

Deehan A, Taylor C, Strang J (1997). The general practitioner, the drug misuser and the alcohol misuser: major differences in general practitioner activity, therapeutic commitment, and shared care proposals. *British Journal of General Practice*, 47, 705–709.

Department of Health (1996). *The Task Force to Review Services for Drug Misusers: Report of an Independent Review of Drug Treatment Services in England*, HMSO, London.

Department of Health and Social Security (1982). *Treatment and Rehabilitation: Report of the Advisory Council on the Misuse of Drugs (ACMD): Central Funding Initiative*, HMSO, London.

Department of Health and Social Security (1984). *Guidelines of Good Practice in the Management of Drug Misuse – Report of a Medical Working Group*. DHSS, London.

Department of Health, Scottish Home and Health Department and Welsh Office (1991). *Drug misuse and dependence: Guidelines on clinical management*, HMSO, London.

Departments of Health (1999). *Drug Misuse and Dependence – Guidelines on Clinical Management*, The Stationery Office, London.

Druglink May/June (1999). New "Orange" guidelines: care or control, 14(3), 4.

Ford C, Ryrie I (2000). A comprehensive package of support to facilitate the treatment of problem drug users in primary care: an evaluation of the training component. *International Journal of Drug Policy*, 11, 387–392.

Gerada C, Tighe J (1999). A review of shared care protocols for the treatment of problem drug use in England, Scotland and Wales. *British Journal of General Practice*, 49, 125–126.

Glanz A, Taylor C (1986). Findings of a national survey on the role of general practitioners in the treatment of opiate misuse: extent of contact. *British Medical Journal*, 293, 427–430.

Gossop M, Marsden J, Stewart, D (1998). *NTORS at One Year: The National Treatment Outcome Research Study. Changes in Substance Use, Health and Criminal Behaviour One Year After Intake*, Department of Health, London.

Greenwood J (1990). Creating a new drug service in Edinburgh. *British Medical Journal*, 300, 587–589.

Groves P, Heuston J, Albery I, Gerada C, Gossop M, Strang J (2000). Managing opiate misusers in primary care: a local study of support and training issues. *Journal of Substance Use*, 5, 227–233.

Gruer L, Wilson P, Scott R, Elliott L, Macleod J, Harden K, Forrester E, Hinshelwood S, McNulty H, Silk P (1997). General practitioner centred scheme for treatment of opiate dependent drug injectors in Glasgow. *British Medical Journal*, 314, 1730–1735.

Hartnoll RL, Mitcheson MC, Battersby A, Brown G, Ellis M, Fleming P, Hedley N (1980). Evaluation of heroin maintenance in a controlled trial. *Archives of General Psychiatry*, 37, 877–884.

HMSO (1965). *Second Brain Report (Inter-Departmental Committee on Drug Addiction): Drug Addiction – 2nd Report*, HMSO, London.

HMSO (1995). *Tackling Drugs Together – A Strategy for England 1995–1998*, HMSO, London.

MacGregor S, Ettore B, Coomber R, Crosier A, Lodge, H (1990) *Drug services in England and the impact of the central funding initiative. Report*, ISDD, London.

Mitcheson M (1994). Drug clinics in the 1970s. In Strang J, Gossop M (eds). *Heroin Addiction and Drug Policy: The British System*, Oxford University Press, Oxford. pp. 178–191.

NHS Executive (1995). *Department of Health Circular. EL (95) 114. Reviewing Shared Care Arrangements for Drug Misusers*.

Pirie K, Ryan C (1999). GPs refuse to take on care of drug users. *Pulse*, June 5, p. 27.

Roberts I, Benbow E, Cairns A (1997). Deaths for accidental drug poisoning in teenagers. Many deaths in known drug misusers will not have been included in study. *British Medical Journal*, 315, 289.

Ryrie I, Ford C, Barjolin JC, Chowdhury R, Roper C (1999). Supporting GPs to manage drug users in general practice: An evaluation of the SMP project. *International Journal of Drug Policy*, 10, 209–221.

Shapiro H (2000). The Wintercomfort: the price of trust. *Druglink*, 10(15), 4–7.

Strang J (1984). Abstinence or abundance – what goal? *British Medical Journal*, 289, 604.

Strang J (1989). A model service: turning the generalist on to drugs. In MacGregor S (ed). *Drugs and British Society*. Routledge, London.

Strang J, Sheridan J, Barber N (1996). Prescribing injectable and oral methadone to opiate addicts: results from the 1995 national postal survey of community pharmacies in England and Wales. *British Medical Journal*, 313, 270–272.

Strang J, Smith M, Spurrell S (1992). The Community Drug Team. *British Journal of Addiction*, 87, 169–178.

Strang J, Marks I, Dawe S, Powell J, Gossop M, Richards D, Gray J (1997). Type of hospital setting and treatment outcome with heroin addicts. Results from a randomised trial. *British Journal of Psychiatry*, 171, 335–339.

Strang J, Clement S (1994). The introduction of community drug teams. Heroin and Drug Policy. In: Strang J, Gossop M (eds) *Heroin Addiction and Drug Policy: The British System*, Oxford University Press, Oxford.

Tantam D, Donmall M, Webster A, Strang J (1993). Do general practitioners and general psychiatrists want to look after drug misusers? Evaluation of a non-specialist treatment policy. *British Journal of General Practice*, 43(376), 470–474.

Walker M (2001). Shared care for opiate substance misusers in Berkshire. *Pharmaceutical Journal*, 266, 547–552.

17

Training for pharmacists about drug misuse: supporting new developments of the role of community pharmacists

David J Temple

INTRODUCTION

In any profession there will be entrepreneurs who are willing to extend their activities. Such "trail blazers" are necessary to show the way for the rank and file of the profession. Often they will have studied the opportunities available to them and will have been working with members of other professions. Some may have undertaken a formal course of training outside the norm for their profession, although this is not often the case. Usually it is their sense of purpose and sheer enthusiasm for what they are doing which carries them through, and they are often therefore at the forefront of professional development.

However, in order to introduce such developments to the majority of the profession, appropriate education and training are essential (Rawlins, 1991). The "trail blazers" will play a crucial role in the development of that training, working with educators from the profession. In order for new recruits into the profession to be able to work within these new developments, changes will be required to the undergraduate curriculum and the preregistration programme. However, it is obvious that relying solely on this approach will mean waiting for a generation to be trained before sufficient numbers of fresh professionals are available to make a real impact on service delivery. Hence existing practitioners need to be re-trained or at least "topped up". Continuing education serves also to support individuals once they have introduced a new service or approach to their clients.

In this context, any development of new roles for pharmacists in dealing with drug misusers will require them to be adequately trained. Likewise, training will help pharmacists to improve existing roles already offered. Training and development clearly go hand in hand, but the quality of training both in terms of content and delivery are crucial in determining outcomes. This is particularly the case where attitudes of pharmacists need to be influenced, for instance to ensure a non-judgemental delivery of service.

The development of services for drug misusers and the expanded demand on such services has put pressure on many community pharmacists to acquire new skills and knowledge, and sometimes a change in attitude. This chapter will look at areas of training and professional development for this field of service provision.

Recommendations of the Advisory Council on the Misuse of Drugs

The UK government's Advisory Council on the Misuse of Drugs (ACMD) investigated the whole area of training of healthcare professionals and others who dealt with drug misusers at the end of the 1980s and their report was published in 1990 (ACMD, 1990). ACMD recognised that the exact levels of information, work on attitudes and skill training which would be required would vary from profession to profession. They put forward a three-tiered approach with all members of a profession receiving basic training in the area of drug misuse, which would include a basic awareness and understanding of the problem. Certain key resource staff would require advanced training and hence be in a position to assist in the training of more junior colleagues. A third tier was restricted to specialist drugs workers who were directly involved in the management of drug-related problems.

ACMD had sought evidence from all relevant professional bodies at the time, including the Royal Pharmaceutical Society of Great Britain (RPSGB). The RPSGB responded that *"pharmacists, in their undergraduate course and in subsequent continuing education, were given a thorough knowledge of the actions and uses of drugs and medicines"*. The RPSGB went on to state that *"pharmacists were 'ideally placed' with subsequent training to offer advice when drugs might be or were being misused"* (ACMD, 1990). The nature of this "subsequent training" was not described. In contrast, ACMD's recommendations were clear, that the approach in training should be primarily person-based rather than substance-based. Furthermore, according to ACMD training should include an opportunity to explore one's own and society's attitudes towards problem drug users.

The specific recommendation to RPSGB was that it should *"urgently review the coverage of drugs and HIV/AIDS in both undergraduate and post-basic training of pharmacists. Specific attention should be paid to the reduction of harm resulting from problem drug use and the patterns and practices of local drugs and HIV/AIDS services"*. Furthermore, *"community pharmacists would benefit greatly from more involvement in multidisciplinary training within their health districts"* (ACMD, 1990).

In the early 1990s two major training initiatives were implemented for community pharmacists. The first was a distance-learning pack comprising an audio tape and ring-binder of print-based information (Daniels, 1992) and the other was a face-to-face training package aimed to support pharmacy-based needle exchange schemes (College of Pharmacy Practice, 1991). The pack, drawing on experience of the Welsh Centre for Postgraduate Pharmaceutical Education, comprised lectures and video footage to stimulate discussion, and attempted to deal with some of the attitudinal issues surrounding drug misuse.

Working Party on pharmaceutical services for drug misusers

In 1998 an RPSGB Working Party reviewed the whole issue of pharmaceutical services for drug misusers (RPSGB, 1998). This provided a broad look at services offered at that time to drug misusers and made a total of 59 recommendations. Many of these suggested changes to the very strict laws governing the dispensing and supply of con-trolled drugs, in order to reflect the massive increase in daily instalment dispensing to drug users over the previous decade. Other recommendations related to good dis-pensing practice, including dispensing of private prescriptions for drug misusers. Practical issues were covered, such as the apparent conflict between confidentiality and the need for sharing information as part of providing a safe and professional serv-ice, the safety of staff and others, and issues around the Misuse of Drugs Regulations (see Chapter 9). Furthermore, it was recommended that pharmacists, not specialist in the field of substance misuse, should not become involved in the direct teaching of children and young people.

Throughout the report there was an undercurrent for the need for training, with seven specific recommendations around training and education. These covered both undergraduate and postgraduate continuing education, including a suggested course content for undergraduates. In its summary the Working Party suggested, as the way forward, that the Government should set up a multi-professional interdepartmental review to urgently address the issues recommended in the report, to ensure that better use is made of the existing network of community pharmacies. Although the report was broadly accepted by the RPSGB Council, in the following years there has been no indication of the Government responding positively to the concept of a review. Likewise, the Council itself has been slow to implement those recommendations which are in its power to enact.

Clinical governance and community pharmacy
More recently the Government has also placed accountability for provision of quality services, via clinical governance, firmly at the heart of all health services (Department of Health, 1999a). Clinical governance can be defined as *"the means by which organ-isations ensure the provision of quality clinical care by making individuals account-able for setting, maintaining and monitoring performance standards"*. One of the key features of clinical governance is the need for clinicians (including pharmacists) to maintain a level of competence through training and professional development in order to provide patient care of high quality according to set standards. For pharmacists involved in providing services for drug misusers the emphasis is on being aware of pharmacists' roles, taking responsibly for maintaining competence, skills, and know-ledge through continuing education and professional development and being part of a risk management structure to ensure safe and effective services.

UNDERGRADUATE EDUCATION AND TRAINING
The RPSGB Working Party report focused on undergraduate education. Following a survey of schools of pharmacy undertaken on behalf of this Working Party in 1997–1998, it emerged that all provided information about legal issues surrounding controlled drugs and the pharmacology of most drugs liable to be misused. However the social aspects of drug misuse, including such areas as government policy, treatment services available and harm reduction approaches were often much less well covered. When covered, this was often only as part of an optional course. The Working Party suggested a detailed undergraduate core course content (see Table 17.1). It was sug-gested that much of this material should be taught in workshop format, to facilitate

discussion of ideas and attitudes and that at least one session should involve a guest lecturer from a local drugs agency. Multi-professional training was also encouraged (RPSGB, 1998). Many of these recommendations are in line with the previous ACMD suggestions (ACMD, 1990).

This report was timely, since all schools of pharmacy were then in the process of introducing a new four-year curriculum. This may have provided an opportunity to look again at the teaching of drug misuse. In particular, schools needed to consider the Working Party's other suggestion, that *"Information about drug dependence and drugs liable to misuse should not simply be provided as an isolated topic, but incorporated into other parts of the undergraduate course, in order to underline the wider perspective of substance misuse and emphasise that drug users often have other health needs, as well as those relating to their drug use"* (RPSGB, 1998).

However, progress in this area is likely to be limited, due to the pressure on the timetable from the more traditional areas of pharmaceutical science. Nonetheless, RPSGB does have an opportunity to press the Working Party's proposals, if it so wishes, during the five-yearly accreditation inspection visit to each school.

A number of methods can be employed to enhance undergraduate education about substance misuse, including the use of multidisciplinary teaching, for example with medical and nursing students. However, multidisciplinary teaching at undergraduate level remains a vexed question in most of the British schools of pharmacy. Very few schools are sited in institutions with schools of medicine or nursing (or where they are, they are on separate campuses) and pressures of the timetable would make joint sessions extremely difficult to organise. Joint lectures may seem attractive from a cost-saving point of view, provided large enough lecture theatre could be found. However, it is highly likely that the two groups would sit on opposite sides of the lecture theatre and not mix at all. The assumption is that the lecture is primarily geared at the other group and hence less relevant to themselves. Small group workshop/discussion periods would be ideal, but unless equal weight was placed on the assessment process for the course unit by both disciplines, one group of students would be tempted to take this approach less seriously and hence impair the experience for the other group. Timetabling and managing a series of such workshops for two or more large course cohorts would be a logistical challenge. However, the concept of involving the local drug team, especially if they employ a pharmacist, is much more realistic. Such sessions must be properly "hosted" by a regular member of staff from the school, to ensure that the content of the session is effectively integrated within the course.

The schools could do well to explore these issues with their own students. Many are eager to learn more in this area, especially to try to understand the situation from the users' point of view. Students in Belfast in the early 1980s organised for the University's Television Production Unit to film interviews between the then Head of School and two injecting drug users. This was at a time when there was very little hard drug misuse in the Province. The video was used for several years as a teaching aid.

Adequate opportunities must be provided within the undergraduate course for students to examine their own attitudes and values in the context of drug misuse and drug misusers. In Strathclyde, for instance, discussion groups based around vignettes of real-life drug users have been introduced. These have been carefully designed with the assistance of a pharmacist working within the Greater Glasgow drug misuse team and allow the students to fully explore a variety of social and other issues and their own personal attitudes, as well as the basic pharmaceutical questions (Coggan, personal communication). Likewise, in Trinity College, Dublin, students are able to visit the local Drug Treatment Centre, where they talk to three to four clients who are at various stages of treatment. This is the key element, because the students realise that drug users are ordinary human beings and not the psychopathic lepers portrayed in the media. There is also a chance to attend an open public meeting of Narcotics Anonymous. As a result of this experience, on qualifying they are much more open to working with drug users in pharmacy-based methadone services (Corrigan, personal communication).

POSTGRADUATE EDUCATION AND TRAINING FOR PHARMACISTS

The RPSGB Working Party recommended that the existing providers of training for practising pharmacists in the field of drug misuse should continue to provide such training and update it at regular intervals. The same overall syllabus (Table 17.1) was recommended for training practising pharmacists (RPSGB, 1998).

The English Centre published a new print-based distance learning pack *Drug Use and Misuse* in 1998 (CPPE, 1998). This pack consisted of two of the now familiar spiral-bound books: part A – Practical issues surrounding drug misuse and the pharmacist: part B – Drugs which are misused. Part B was an update of the traditional approach to teaching in this area, but refreshingly does include separate chapters on anabolic steroids, volatile solvents and alcohol. However, part A does attempt to provide some answers as to why people take drugs, current principles for the treatment of drug dependence, including stimulant dependence, and medical complications of injecting drug use. The final section addresses issues around syringe and needle exchange schemes in pharmacies. However, there is little challenge to pharmacists' pre-existing attitudes to drug users.

In contrast, a pack from the Scottish Centre for Post Qualification Pharmaceutical Education (SCPPE) – *Pharmaceutical Care of the Drug Misuser*, published in early 1999 (SCPPE, 1999) – does attempt to change attitudes of pharmacists towards drug users. There is a clear attempt to help pharmacists to see the issue from the user's point of view. In the first part, which deals with "understanding the drug user", it makes the valid point that "there is no such thing as the typical drug user". The first module reviews the family circumstances, health, employment and housing situation of the drug users interviewed in an extensive survey of Scottish drug users. Separate sections explore their expectations of agencies and services available to them, including factors influencing their choice of a pharmacy. This leads to a discussion of services available from pharmacies and users' views of good and bad aspects of those services, and highlights the aspect of greater privacy and the quality of advice given.

The second part of this pack relates specifically to harm minimisation and the prevention of viral infection, with a brief section on methadone maintenance therapy. As such it builds on earlier packs from the Scottish Centre on syringe and needle exchange (SCPPE, 1995) and aspects of methadone prescribing (SCPPE, 1996). Both were produced specifically at the request of and with funding from the Scottish Office, to support schemes then in their infancy in Scotland. The methadone pack was particularly well received and was adopted in other areas (for instance North Wales H.A.) as an obligatory requirement for

Table 17.1 Suggested course content covering pharmacists' needs for education and training in the area of drug misuse (adapted from RPSGB, 1998)

Subject	Examples of content
Dependence and addiction	Both physical and psychological and the difference between drug misuse and drug dependence.
Drugs which are misused	Illicit, over-the-counter and prescription medicines, and the manner of misuse.
Psychopharmacology	The psychopharmacology of drugs liable to misuse.
Legislation	Including not just prescribing (Misuse of Drugs Regulations), but also offences under the Misuse of Drugs Act and the different penalties imposed for offences relating to the different classes of drugs.
Service provision	What the services are, how they are organised, relevant recent legislation and known levels of drug misuse.
Treatment	How client assessments are made, and substitute prescribing. Special emphasis should be given to treatment philosophies, such as why methadone maintenance should not necessarily be deemed a failure, focusing on issues relating to harm reduction in the light of HIV infection and hepatitis B and C.
Pharmacists' roles	Needle exchange and the supervision of self-administration of prescribed medication, and how the pharmacist fits in with other health professionals working with the client.
Social skills	How to maintain a non-judgmental attitude towards service users, how to become proactive and when to step in with advice.
Harm reduction/minimisation	The role of harm minimisation/reduction and its impact on the nature of drug services.
Other treatments	Motivational interviewing, cognitive-behaviour therapy. Brief overviews of such approaches would be useful and would help the pharmacist to appreciate more fully the work undertaken with clients by their local drug services. This is essential if we are to work closely with other professionals in this area.

pharmacists joining their scheme to offer a service of supervised consumption of methadone on the premises (Morgan D, personal communication).

The RPSGB Working Party made other recommendations for continuing education of pharmacists. With regard to practising pharmacists, there should be more opportunities for multidisciplinary training with other local professionals who deal with specific aspects of drug misuse. This has been a feature of face-to-face courses on HIV/drug misuse in Wales throughout the 1990s (Temple, 1996).

An innovative training session was held in West Wales in 1998 instigated by the Health Authority, in collaboration with WCPPE. This was a prelude to a local methadone consumption scheme and attracted a joint audience of doctors and pharmacists. The day started with a presentation from a local theatre group designed to explore participants' stereotypical views of drug users. They went on to present in theatrical style a "typical" life story, which had been developed in collaboration with a local Community Drug Team. The actors remained "in character" and were open to questions from the pharmacists and GPs present. This was followed by more traditional lecture-format presentations, but the event provided plenty of opportunities for both sets of professionals to debate in depth the practicalities of the methadone consumption scheme from their own viewpoint, resulting in greater understanding of the issues all round (personal observations of the author).

In other parts of the UK, multidisciplinary training has been employed for professionals involved in shared care arrangements for managing drug misusers (see Chapter 16). In these situations GPs, pharmacists and members of specialist drug teams all attend training events together, providing an opportunity for team building, problem solving and getting to understand the respective roles of each professional group.

For those pharmacists who wish to become more specialised in this field, a number of diploma and Masters degree courses exist in the UK, providing more in-depth academic education, whilst also providing students with the opportunity to observe clinical specialists working with clients in a number of different clinical settings. Pharmacists receiving such qualifications would be well placed to become "specialist pharmacists" working within drug clinics or advising at health authority/health board level.

The concept of support for the individual pharmacist has already been raised. This needs to be addressed for any pharmacy-based service to drug misusers to be successful. In Wales it has been reported that the more successful syringe and needle exchange schemes have been maintained in those counties where a central link person has been identified, who visits all pharmacies in the scheme acting as mentor and providing training (Temple 1996). The example in Leicestershire, where a pharmacist has been employed for the past decade by the community drug team, has been commended by the ACMD in their report *AIDS and Drug Misuse Update* (ACMD, 1993). More recently, the supervised methadone scheme in Glasgow has been highlighted as good practice in the Government's 10-year strategy document *Tackling Drugs to Build a Better Britain* (The Stationery Office, 1998). This scheme relies heavily on the supporting role of a pharmacist employed by the Health Board.

A CURRICULUM FOR SUBSTANCE MISUSE?

At an undergraduate level, there is a need for a curriculum which covers the knowledge, attitude and skills which pharmacists will require in order to be able to work competently and empathetically with drug misusers – see Table 17.1. However, such a curriculum needs to be adopted by all schools of pharmacy.

For postgraduate education and training, there may be a need for a curriculum to be developed which enables pharmacists to provide services for drug users in the context of clinical governance and as part of local drug services. Pharmacy is not alone in this. All healthcare professions have recognised the need for training in this area. For instance the medical profession in a report from the British Medical Association (British Medical Association, 1997) has stated that "*all doctors have a responsibility to understand the basis of the aetiology, life histories and recognised treatments for this group of patients and how this impinges on their practice*". One could also develop the theme of the new Government clinical guidelines (Departments of Health 1999b). This defines doctors as "generalists" providing basic services, "specialised generalists" providing a higher degree of services and requiring a higher level of training and expertise, and offering peer support to generalists and "specialists" whose work is usually within a drug clinic, whose expertise is of the highest level, and whose clients are likely to be the most complex cases. This mirrors the earlier ACMD (1990) concept. By direct analogy, training and education could be developed for pharmacists at each of these three levels.

CONCLUSIONS

The massive increase in the incidence and complexity of drug misuse in the UK over the past two decades has coincided with the recognition of HIV, hepatitis B and C and other blood-borne viruses as risks to injecting users (Department of Health, 1996). At the same time the pharmacy profession has undergone a major re-examination of itself, commencing with the Nuffield Report, moving through various initiatives leading to the "Pharmacy in a New Age" concept. New and "extended roles" for pharmacists have been recognised, including the area of services to drug users. Changes in the undergraduate curriculum, such as those suggested by the RPSGB Working Party Report, are necessary but will take more than a generation to bring real change into every day practice. Changing existing practice will depend on continuing education opportunities and pharmacists' full involvement in the continuing professional development process. Important constructive recommendations for improved training have been made. But recommendations are not enough: the acid test will be the extent to which real changes in basic and supplementary training are actually introduced and maintained. Only in this way will pharmacists be able to embrace the breadth of their role within the substance misuse field in a positive, supportive and effective manner, and feel both competent and confident in working with drug users and in partnerships with other members of the health care team.

REFERENCES

Advisory Council on the Misuse of Drugs (1990). *Problem Drug Use: A Review of Training, The Advisory Council on the Misuse of Drugs* HMSO, London.
Advisory Council on the Misuse of Drugs (1993). *AIDS and Drug Misuse Update, The Advisory Council on the Misuse of Drugs*, HMSO, London.
British Medical Association (1997). *The Misuse of Drugs – a report by the British Medical Association*. Harwood Academic Publishers, Amsterdam.
Centre for Postgraduate Pharmaceutical Education (1998). *Drug use and misuse*, The Centre for Pharmacy Postgraduate Education, University of Manchester.

College of Pharmacy Practice (1991). *Prevention of AIDS: a pharmacist, role (Training Pack),* College of Pharmacy Practice, Coventry.

Daniels VG (1992). *Treatment of Drug Dependence: A Training Manual for Pharmacists,* Centre for Pharmacy Postgraduate Education, Manchester.

Department of Health (1996*). The Task Force to Review Services for Drug Misusers: Report of an Independent Review of Drug Treatment Services in England,* Department of Health, London.

Department of Health (1999a). *A First-Class Service: Quality in the New NHS,* The Stationery Office, London.

Department of Health (1999b). *Drug Misuse and Dependence Guidelines on Clinical Management,* The Stationery office, London.

Rawlins MD (1991). Extending the role of the community pharmacist depends on extending training and regulation. *British Medical Journal,* 302, 427–428.

RPSGB (1998). *Report of the Working Party on Pharmaceutical Services for Drug Misusers,* RPSGB, London.

SCPPE (1995). *Syringe and needle exchange.* Scottish Centre for Post Qualification Pharmaceutical Education, Strathclyde University, Glasgow.

SCPPE (1996). *Pharmaceutical aspects of methadone prescribing.* Scottish Centre for Post Qualification Pharmaceutical Education, Strathclyde University, Glasgow.

SCPPE (1999) *Pharmaceutical care of the drug misuser.* Scottish Centre for Post Qualification Pharmaceutical Education, Strathclyde University, Glasgow.

Temple DJ (1996). Reflections on the development of pharmacy-based syringe and needle exchange schemes in Wales. In: Phillips SA, Temple DJ and Delamont S (Eds.). *Qualitative Research in Pharmacy Practice,* Avebury Press, Aldershot, pp. 129–151.

The Stationery Office (1998). *Tackling Drugs to build a Better Britain: The Government's 10-Year Strategy for Tackling Drug Misuse. Guidance Notes,* The Stationery Office, London.

18

The way forward – greater specialism or more generalism?

Janie Sheridan and John Strang

Community pharmacy has long been an important part of the addictions treatment response in the UK. The substance misuse field has seen many changes over the last two decades, including the way the focus on treatment of drug users has oscillated between primary and secondary care. However, regardless of where responsibility has rested for treatment, responsibility for the delivery of medication to patients has rested almost exclusively with the community pharmacist. With the exception of a few specialist drug clinics which dispense methadone and other drugs on-site, community pharmacists in the UK dispense all other prescriptions for drugs such as methadone, often in daily instalments, and more recently with supervised consumption at the pharmacy. Furthermore, as with most areas of health care, community pharmacy has also seen many changes, and in the last 15 years community pharmacists have been willing to involve themselves in an increasingly wide range of services such as needle and syringe exchange, dispensing methadone prescriptions, and most recently in the supervision of administration of methadone on the pharmacy premises.

The 1999 government Clinical Guidelines (Departments of Health, 1999) recognised the vital role that community pharmacy plays in the delivery of treatment. However, in some ways the Guidelines go one step further and recognise that community pharmacists are an integral part of any team of health professionals who manage drug misusers. To this end, pharmacists themselves may now start to see themselves more and more involved as partners in shared care arrangements.

One example of this is the "4-Way Agreement" model of shared care that operates in West Berkshire, and is now being adopted by many other areas (Walker, 2001). In this arrangement (developed by a local pharmacist), the GP, the specialist service, the pharmacist and the "client" all enter into an agreement which defines their roles and responsibilities. One of the main benefits from such an arrangement has been that avenues of communication which have previously been underutilised, such as that between the GP and the pharmacist, are now seen as "normal" and indeed a vital part of service provision. This shared care arrangement works to agreed protocols, which are designed to maximise the safety and efficiency of treatment, whilst minimising problems and indeed identifying issues and resolving them before they reach the problem stage.

But it is not just in the area of "shared care" where pharmacy has expanded its role in terms of working with drug users. In several areas of the UK, a pharmacist is employed as a specialist to develop, advise and manage pharmacy services for drug users. An example of this has been in Glasgow, Scotland, where the post of Area Pharmacy Specialist – Drug Misuse has been in existence since the mid-1990s (see Chapter 5). In hospital clinics, specialist pharmacists have sometimes been employed by drug dependency clinics to manage their in-house dispensary, from which methadone is dispensed to clients who consume it under the supervision of the pharmacist. The expertise of such specialist pharmacists can, and has been, utilised in other areas such as the development of in-house protocols for the prescribing and dispensing of drugs such as lofexidine and buprenorphine, and for the development of dose assessment clinics, overdose prevention interventions and the more appropriate management of co-existing over-the-counter misuse problems. The traditional skills of audit have also been utilised in the evaluation of prescribing regimes. Many of these specialist pharmacists have come to the drug dependency clinics from a community pharmacy background, bringing with them expertise gained whilst providing primary care services for drug users.

Pharmacists have also moved into the addictions field in positions such as needle exchange co-ordinators, and it is likely that, in the future, pharmacists may also find themselves in posts such as shared care co-ordinators, working across the interface between GPs and specialist clinics.

However, while many pharmacists may wish to move into more specialised roles, other pharmacists will wish to remain in the rich arena of primary care, providing services to whole communities from their pharmacies – communities which include drug users and those directly and indirectly affected by drug misuse. Such practitioners can rest assured that there is an increasingly solid evidence base for much of the treatment. Studies have shown that treatment is effective in producing positive benefits at many levels – health gain, reduction in injecting, reduction in involvement in acquisitive crime, for example (Gossop *et al.*, 2000). There is, however, a continual rise in the numbers of people seeking drug treatment and consequently in the demand for community pharmacy services.

At some point, it is possible that those who are heavily involved in service provision to drug users may become overwhelmed by this demand, and disillusioned by the lack of support from their peers, who may choose not to involve themselves in this area of practice. The Government's new Clinical Guidelines remind doctors of the GMC's statement that "It is unethical for a doctor to withhold treatment from a patient on the basis of a moral judgement that the patient's activities or lifestyles might have contributed to the condition for which treatment is being sought". The Guidelines go on to state that "All individuals are entitled to the same standard of care and range of treatments, as set out in these Guidelines" (Departments of Health, 1999). Whilst these statements are directed at doctors, it is appropriate to extrapolate this to all primary health care professionals who work within the NHS and wider healthcare field.

Another aspect of the Department of Health's Guidelines can also usefully be considered from the point of view of the community pharmacist. The Guidelines have suggested three levels of doctor practitioner: the *generalist* – a doctor who may be involved in caring for, and the provision of general medical care to, drug users, but for whom it is not their main area of work; the *specialised generalist* who has a special interest and expertise in working with this group of patients within their wider practice; and the *specialist* whose particular specialist area of work is drug misuse and who probably works in a dedicated clinic (Departments of Health, 1999). As pharmacists are increasingly recognised as key colleagues in the provision of medical care for drug users, one could envisage a similar "classification" of pharmacists, with training being made available to ensure that pharmacists at each level are appropriately skilled, knowledgeable and confident to provide services at that level.

On the basis of this new terminology, the *generalist pharmacist* would be a term which related to all community pharmacists including those for whom their involvement with drug services may be no more than dispensing prescriptions for a small number of methadone patients, or occasionally supplying injecting equipment to injectors. A general grounding in drug misuse services, harm reduction philosophies, risks associated with drug misuse and a knowledge of methadone prescribing and dispensing would seem the key basic areas in which such pharmacists would need to be competent. *Specialised generalist pharmacists* would be those who were more significantly involved – for example, providing a needle exchange service and/or dispensing methadone prescriptions to a larger number of patients and for whom contact with drug services would be a regular occurrence. Such pharmacists would be expected to have additional skills and a more in-depth knowledge of the field. For *specialist pharmacists*, such as those who might work at drug clinics, their levels of knowledge, skills and competence would need to be substantially greater, and would probably have involved undertaking diplomas and MSc courses in addiction-related subjects. These specialist pharmacists would also provide expert professional consultation services to community pharmacists and others about local initiatives which include particular pharmacy components.

Support for pharmacists in terms of training is not without resource implications and the impact of trained pharmacists will only be maximised once they are recognised as part of the care team, their skills being valued and utilised as they work in appropriate partnerships. Such recommendations will need the backing of the profession, the willingness of individual practitioners and the backing of primary care teams and health authorities.

REFERENCES

Departments of Health (1999). *Drug Misuse and Dependence: Guidelines on Clinical Management*, London The Stationery Office.

Gossop M, Marsden J, Stewart D, Rolfe A (2000). Reductions in acquisitive crime and drug use after treatment of addiction problems: 1-year follow-up outcomes. *Drug and Alcohol Dependence*, 58, 165–172.

Walker M (2001). Shared care for opiate substance misusers in Berkshire. *Pharmaceutical Journal*, 266, 547–552.

Further reading

Advisory Council on the Misuse of Drugs (2000). *Reducing Drug-Related Deaths: A Report by the Advisory Council on the Misuse of Drugs.* The Stationery Office, London.

Berridge VS (1999). *Opium and the People.* Free Association Books Ltd: London.

Department of Health (2000). *Pharmacy in a new age: A programme for pharmacy in the National Health Service.* Department of Health, London.

Departments of Health *et al.* (1999). *Drug Misuse and Dependence: Guidelines on Clinical Management,* The Stationery Office: London.

Derricott J, Preston A, Hunt N (1999). *Safer Injecting Briefing.* HIT, Liverpool.

EMCDDA (2000). *Insights No 3. Reviewing current practice in drug-substitution treatment in the European Union.*

Gossop M, Marsden J, Stewart D (2001). *NTORS After Five Years. The National Treatment Outcome Research Study.* National Addiction Centre, London.

Holloway SWF (1991). *Royal Pharmaceutical Society of Great Britain 1841 to 1991: A Political and Social History.* Pharmaceutical Press, London.

Miller W, Rollnick S (1991). *Motivational Interviewing: Preparing to Change Addictive Behaviour,* Guilford Press, New York.

Preston A (1996). *The Methadone Briefing,* Andrew Preston/ISDD, London.

Royal College of Psychiatry and Physicians (2000). *Drug Dilemmas and Choices,* Gaskell, London.

RPSGB (1998). *Report of the Working Party on Pharmaceutical Services for Drug Misusers: A Report to the Council of the Royal Pharmaceutical Society of Great Britain.* London.

Sievewright N (2000). *Community Treatment of Drug Misuse: More Than Methadone.* Cambridge University Press, Cambridge.

Tackling Drugs to Build a Better Britain: The Government's Ten-Year Strategy for Tackling Drugs (Cm 3945) (1998), The Stationery Office, London.

Ward J, Mattick RP, Hall W (1998). *Methadone Maintenance Treatment and Other Opioid Replacement Therapies.* Harwood Academic: Australia.

Wills S (1997). *Drugs of Abuse,* Pharmaceutical Press, London.

Index